From Company Doctors
to Managed Care

To Chuck,

In solidarity,

Isaac

From **Company Doctors** to **Managed Care**

The United Mine Workers' Noble Experiment

Ivana Krajcinovic

ILR Press
an imprint of
Cornell University Press
Ithaca and London

Cornell Studies in Industrial and Labor Relations No. 31

First published 1997 by Cornell University Press

Printed in the United States of America

Library of Congress Cataloging-in-Publication Data

Krajcinovic, Ivana, b. 1965
    From company doctors to managed care : the United Mine Workers'
noble experiment / Ivana Krajcinovic.
        p.   cm. — (Cornell studies in industrial and labor relations ;
no. 31)
    Includes bibliographical references.
    ISBN 0-8014-3392-4 (cloth : alk. paper)
    1. United Mine Workers of America. Welfare and Retirement Fund.
2. Miners—Medical care—United States. 3. Insurance, Health—
United States. 4. Collective bargaining—Mining, industry—United
States. I. Title. II. Series.
RA413.7.M55K73   1997   97-15098
362.1'088'622—dc21

Cornell University Press strives to utilize environmentally responsible
suppliers and materials to the fullest extent possible in the publishing
of its books. Such materials include vegetable-based, low-VOC inks
and acid-free papers that are also either recycled, totally chlorine-free,
or party composed of nonwood fibers.

Cloth printing   10 9 8 7 6 5 4 3 2 1

for my parents
Dusan & Tanya

proceeds from the sale of this book go to
The Frontier Strike Fund, Las Vegas &
The Federation of University Employees Strike Fund, Yale University
¡Sí, se puede!

Contents

Figures, Tables, and Maps

Figures

Tables

Maps

Abbreviations

AFL	American Federation of Labor
AMA	American Medical Association
AMO	Area Medical Office
ARHI	Appalachian Regional Hospitals, Inc.
BCOA	Bituminous Coal Operators Association
CIO	Congress of Industrial Organizations
The Fund	UMWA Welfare and Retirement Fund
Fund Archives	The UMWA Health and Retirement Funds Archives, West Virginia and Regional History Collection, West Virginia University Library, Morgantown
HMO	Health Maintenance Organization
ILGWU	International Ladies' Garment Workers' Union
Lorin Edgar Kerr papers	Lorin Edgar Kerr papers, Manuscripts and Archives, Yale University, New Haven
MMHA	Miners Memorial Hospital Association
Robert Kaplan papers	Robert Kaplan papers, Manuscripts and Archives, Yale University, New Haven
UAW	United Automobile, Aircraft, and Agricultural Implement Workers
UMWA	United Mine Workers of America

Acknowledgments

I began this project in 1990, almost exactly at the same time as I began my involvement in union organizing. Through the subsequent years, I strayed further and further from scholarly pursuits toward becoming a full-time organizer. It is with a certain sense of irony, therefore, that I offer this work at the same time as I have adopted a vocation that is about as far from the academic world as can be imagined.

On a deeper level, however, I truly believe that this work profited from the exposure I have had to unions. There is no issue more central to organizing in the 1990s than health care. This realization strengthened my commitment to studying the origin of collectively bargained health plans and the particularly visionary plan created by the UMWA. At the same time, my work as an organizer has enabled me to understand the complex interplay of union power, industry conditions, and the desire of both employers and unions to capture worker loyalty.

Having been fortunate, then, to benefit from both the world of scholars and the world of trade unionists, I have two groups of people to thank. The foundation of this book owes an enormous debt to David Weiman and Jody Sindelar. This project also benefited from comments made by Alan Derickson and Ed Berkowitz. David Montgomery provided valuable insights and wise advice throughout, and has remained an inspiration for his ability to combine unparalleled scholarship and relevant activism.

Never will I be able to repay fully the members of HERE Locals 34 and 35 at Yale University for their unconditional support of the Graduate Employees and Students Organization. Half the proceeds from the sale of this book go to their strike fund as a gesture of support for the people who really work to make Yale a better place. I also want to thank HERE for allowing me to join the fight for justice in the service industry. In particular, I'd like to thank the staff at Local 2850 for putting up with me while writing this book and attempting to climb out of the ivory tower.

My good friend Chris Nelson produced the wonderful maps included here. Finally, Fran Benson provided the enthusiasm I needed to finish this project. Fran asked all the right questions, and I hope I have done her insights justice by providing the right answers.

I. K.

From Company Doctors
to Managed Care

The Centrality of Health Benefits in Labor Contracts

A pivotal issue in contemporary health care debates is the provision of affordable care, especially to low-income and high-risk groups that historically have been denied access to quality care. The variety of structures of health care financing and delivery systems in the United States provides different incentives for the provision of cost-effective quality care. While most attention has been paid to private and government-sponsored health care systems, almost no attention has been afforded to health care plans that arise out of collective bargaining. One such system, the Welfare and Retirement Fund of the United Mine Workers of America (UMWA) provides one of the most innovative and important examples of alternative health care systems capable of providing affordable care to a high-risk population.

The Welfare and Retirement Fund (the Fund) was a novelty when it was established by the UMWA in the 1940s. It emerged out of a collective bargaining process which transferred financing to the employers and control of the plan to the union; it provided a level of quality of care that surpassed not only what previously had been available in the coalfields but also what was commonly available throughout most of the United States; and it departed significantly from conventional health care delivery and reimbursement mechanisms by employing group practices, managed care, treatment review, closed panels, and retainer payments. The Fund was also used, as perhaps no other item on the collective bargaining agenda, to transform industrial and labor relations in the coal fields.

What the UMWA pioneered in the decades after the Second World War has now become the norm. Health benefits are a standard feature of labor contracts, providing the most common form of access to quality health care. The advent of health maintenance organizations and preferred provider organizations has increased the popularity of the delivery and reimbursement methods promoted by the Fund. Negotiations over the extent and type of health care coverage have become a contentious bargaining issue and the most frequent cause of labor disputes.

The experience of the Fund should be of interest to both scholars and policymakers in the fields of health care and labor. Health care policymakers and scholars can draw valuable lessons from the Fund's design and implementation of its innovations in health care provision. Three decades of experience provide a means to evaluate these innovations with an eye toward the further refinement of their contemporary descendants. Most notably, the Fund's experience shows the benefits of closed panels of providers and retainer payments in providing cost-effective care. The manner in which the Fund implemented and maintained these programs is also instructive as it avoided the rigid, third-party cost control that is criticized vociferously by contemporary providers. Fund review of physicians and hospitals was based instead on comprehensive evaluation and education of providers done locally by administrators who were themselves physicians.

The Fund would have experienced even greater financial returns to its programs had it not had to contend with a progressively sicker and aging beneficiary pool. Changes in coal production following the war heightened the incidence of respiratory illness and mining injuries while concurrently producing an older workforce. At first glance these trends may appear to limit the evaluation and applicability of the Fund's results. In fact, these changes in the needs of Fund beneficiaries are consistent with trends that are becoming increasingly evident in the United States as the population ages and the toll of diseases like AIDS and cancer places tremendous burdens on health care systems.

The Fund's experience also illuminates the challenges posed by providing care in underserved areas. The experience of Fund beneficiaries is similar to that of inner-city Medicaid recipients and residents of rural areas because of their socioeconomic backgrounds, health needs, and access to health care providers. The Fund overcame numerous obstacles to achieve enormous success in caring for a demographically similar group. In fact, the Fund's success may have been due, in part, to the very underdevelopment of the mining regions. As a dominant provider and financier of health care, the Fund achieved a degree of control that facilitated the promotion of its innovations.

Labor historians and labor relations experts can examine the UMWA's experience with the Fund to better understand the centrality of health benefits as a collective bargaining issue. Bargaining for benefits is a relatively recent phenomenon, yet has become a defining issue of labor contracts and labor disputes in the post-World War II era. Health benefits are central in part because they are tremendously expensive to provide and, as such, compete with other economic items on collective bargaining agendas. The importance of health benefits also stems from their role in defining the place of unions and employers in the eyes of workers. In a society without universal coverage, workers are likely to be loyal to parties that provide health care. Employers see the returns to loyalty in terms of greater productivity while unions see these returns in the form of greater solidarity. Both the cost of health benefits and the returns to loyalty have made health care an important bargaining chip in the postwar era. As such, since the 1940s the provision of health care has been used to fashion some of the most far-reaching compromises between labor and management. The Fund provides not only one of the earliest and most extensive examples of the dynamics of the bargaining process, but also the clearest example of the consequences of such compromises.

It will be tempting for those interested in labor to read only those sections focusing on labor issues, and for those interested in health care to read only those sections pertaining primarily to health. But to do so would be to miss the point. Those interested in collective bargaining need to understand the potential contributions of health care innovations to the costs of contracts. Otherwise, given the nature of unfettered health care cost escalation, bargaining is destined to be reduced simply to demanding greater resources to maintain health benefits. These resources can only be devoted to health care at the expense of other economic items and, ultimately, at the expense of the competitiveness of union firms. By the same token, those interested in health care need to understand that innovations in health care are ultimately subject to the dictates of collective bargaining. Health care policymakers may not always have the time and resources to maximize the contribution of even the most valiant efforts at reform. They may also find that they must accommodate political objectives that are at odds with health policy goals.

An examination of innovations in health care provision and the exigencies of collective bargaining in tandem sheds further light on key Fund decisions. The UMWA's leaders allowed Fund administrators great latitude in designing pathbreaking reforms because they were convinced that the formidable needs of their beneficiaries could only be met if they were cared for cost effectively. Yet UMWA leaders also insisted on ensuring that the Fund would provide high profile care that would cement the loyalty of its members. Fund administrators therefore prioritized the provision of hospital and specialist care—and even built a set of Fund hospitals—as a concession to those political needs, despite the fact that this bias was inconsistent with their other policy objectives.

To appreciate fully the need to examine jointly the UMWA's innovations in health care provision and in collective bargaining, the larger context of changing industry conditions during the 1940s should also be considered.

The competitiveness of union coal proved to be the major impetus behind the political compromises that shaped the Fund's health care policy innovations. The real and projected fortunes of union coal determined, in large part, the fortunes of the Fund. Downturns in the industry cut short some of the Fund's most well-intentioned actions and prompted some of the most cynical manipulations of Fund policy.

Indeed, changes in industry conditions laid bare the inherent tension between health care objectives and political compromises fashioned by the UMWA. Faced with rising competition from alternate fuels and nonunion coal, union president John L. Lewis agreed not to oppose mechanization in the mines in exchange for the ability to provide quality cradle-to-grave services for union members through the Fund. Yet mechanization dramatically altered the health needs of Fund beneficiaries. Mechanization resulted in layoffs and also reduced the number of new hires, thereby initiating an aging of the mining workforce. Concurrently, mechanization increased the hazards in the mines by elevating dust and noise levels. As miners inhaled more dust they were more likely to develop respiratory illnesses. Higher noise levels diminished miners' ability to listen for stresses in the mine roofs, thereby increasing the injury rates associated with roof falls. The resultant older and sicker workforce would have been better served had the Fund promoted greater attention to the prevention of occupational illness and injury and placed greater emphasis on primary care. However, this approach would have violated the political objectives of UMWA leaders. Prevention of occupational hazards would have unacceptably impeded productivity in the mines, while an emphasis on preventive medicine would not have delivered returns to loyalty as great as those provided by relatively more glamorous hospital and specialist care.

In retrospect, the failure of Fund administrators and UMWA leaders to recognize and attempt to accommodate the tension between the union's health policy and collective bargaining objectives brought an end to many Fund policies. Visionary at its inception, the Fund ultimately fell victim to the shortsightedness of the union's leaders. Despite its eventual demise, the Fund's legacy remains that of a standard-bearer for an unprecedented manner of providing health care that stands without equal even today. Embracing the challenge of serving a neglected group of workers and their families, the Fund used hitherto untested policies to construct a system of care that focused on access and quality without losing sight of costs. In doing so, the Fund's "noble experiment," in the words of Albert Deutsch, provides lessons that go beyond the collective bargaining arena.

CHAPTER ONE

The Early History of Health Plans for Workers

*T*hroughout the history of worker health plans, unions and employers have been motivated by a few central reasons to promote employment-linked health care. Providing health care allows unions to improve the standard of living of their members and allows employers to achieve greater employee productivity. Moreover, both management and unions recognize that supplying enduring quality care increases workers' attachment to the provider of the benefit. Anxious to garner the returns to greater loyalty as industrialization took hold in the United States, both unions and employers initiated numerous efforts to supply health benefits to workers.

Workers first received benefits linked to health in the late nineteenth century through their own organizations. Most of these early attempts were designed to compensate for lost wages due to illness or injury and were fairly limited and short-lived. By the early twentieth century, employers began offering similarly limited health care plans to workers. Both employers and unions, however, considered health plans to be expendable during economic downturns. The Depression definitively eliminated most worker health plans outside of the company doctor system operating in isolated areas. The efforts of management and labor prior to World War II resulted in few enduring comprehensive health plans with the result that neither side realized an appreciable increase in worker attachment through the provision of these benefits. This failure would help inspire labor and management to adopt a different approach during the 1940s.

Worker health plans reappeared during World War II in a manner that ensured their permanence as unions and employers abandoned attempts to provide health care for workers separately and, instead, negotiated plans through the collective bargaining process. Negotiations determined which party would control and shape the benefits and, hence, reap the returns to increased worker attachment. A few unions like the UMWA were able to establish independent plans which allowed them to adapt coverage to the needs of members and firmly associate the union with the health plan.

Miners always have occupied a unique place in the history of the U.S. labor movement. Concentrated in remote company towns, employed in an industry central to the economy, and displaying a remarkable degree of cohesion within their union and their communities, miners have received the attention of scholars as much for the singularity of their position as for their contribution to the development of the labor movement. The experience of the health plan sponsored by their union, the UMWA, is interesting for these same reasons. Prior to the 1940s, miners were one of the few groups of workers to receive continuous, albeit substandard, health care through the uncommon company doctor system. The UMWA was one of the first unions to take advantage of conditions created by World War II to bargain for employer-financed health benefits to replace the company doctor system. Spurning convention, the UMWA not only retained control over the provision of health benefits, but also utilized then unorthodox managed care principles in arranging for the care of its members. In less than a decade, the Welfare and Retirement Fund they created brought mining families from the backwater to the forefront of medical care.

The experience of the Fund is better understood when evaluated in the context of other health plans developed for workers.[1] An examination of the factors that distinguished the mining industry from other sectors of the economy shows in part why the UMWA created an independent plan markedly different from any other contemporary health plan. Yet the peculiarities of the industry did not alone determine the degree of the Fund's departure from mainstream organization of the provision of medical care. The union's leadership consciously chose to develop an independent plan despite the trend of other unions to choose rapidly maturing commercial plans. UMWA president John L. Lewis would realize what was surely the dream of every labor leader in the immediate postwar era when he captured control of a central benefit and, in doing so, secured the loyalty of his membership.

Labor-Sponsored Health Plans

Prior to the eventual achievement of health plans for workers in the postwar period, unions made various attempts to provide some form of security in the event of illness or injury as a way of securing worker loyalty. Increased cohesiveness of its membership became critical as organized labor sought to increase its presence during the expansion of the economy after the Civil War. During the last three decades of the nineteenth century, the burgeoning trade union movement began offering benefit plans as a mechanism for stabilizing its membership rolls. During a time of frequent economic downturns that reduced wages and employment, unions found it critical to keep members from neglecting to pay dues. A growing body of evidence suggested that workers who received benefits from their unions were more likely to maintain their membership in their unions.[2]

However compelling this logic may have been, true health care benefits were prohibitively expensive and difficult to administer. In practice most unions could offer only limited benefits during this period. At first unions typically provided only death benefits and later added compensation for lost wages during periods of illness and injury. The most common arrangements for medical care were restricted to treatment for specific diseases. In 1892, the International Typographical Union established facilities for members suffering from tuberculosis.[3] Likewise, the best-known direct service clinic, the International Ladies' Garment Workers' Union (ILGWU) New York Health Center was established initially as a clinic to diagnose tuberculosis.

The Western Federation of Miners provided one striking exception to unions' inability to supply medical care. The hardrock miners' union founded more than 20 hospitals across the United States and Canada in the late nineteenth and early twentieth centuries. The hospitals were almost exclusively financed, planned, and governed by the miners themselves and filled a dire need for care in an industry with a high degree of occupational hazard. However admirable, all but three of the hospitals were closed by 1920, victims of periodic economic downturns and depletions of veins of ore that shrank the hospitals' income sources.[4]

By 1930, comprehensive medical plans were offered by only a handful of unions: the Mine, Mill, and Smelter union in Colorado; the letter carriers union in New York City; the public utility workers' union in Milwaukee; the engravers and printers' union in Washington, D.C.; and various locals in Los Angeles.[5] Coverage was somewhat more complete in large urban areas where workers lived in geographically concentrated areas. For example, in the early part of the twentieth century, New York City trade unions covered 20,000 workers in health plans, or 12 percent of the overall U.S. population covered by health insurance.[6]

Not only were the vast majority of labor-sponsored plans limited in scope, but they also were not financially viable in the long term. Most plans were set up on a pay-as-you-go basis and were not based on sound actuarial principles.[7] This meant that the endurance of health plans was linked intimately to the strength of the individual industry and that of the economy in general. As a result, unions typically abandoned health plans in economic downturns, precisely when they were most useful in maintaining membership lists.

Throughout the late nineteenth and early twentieth centuries, health plans were a prohibitively expensive way to increase worker solidarity and, hence, remained a low priority for unions. Moreover, unions discovered a potential conflict between their welfare and employment goals.[8] If unions were to provide extensive benefits to members, they often had to do so by limiting the number of people who could receive them. Furthermore, the conflict between welfare and employment goals was exacerbated over time as the labor movement grew to include poorly paid industrial workers. Low dues were a prerequisite for attracting these workers to the union.[9] In comparison to the staple issues of wages, job security, and the actual survival of unions, health plans were a luxury benefit that would have to wait for better times.

Employer-Sponsored Health Plans

Employers sponsored most of the efforts to provide health care for workers in the period before World War II. The most common incarnation of employer-sponsored care, the ubiquitous company doctor system, arose in high-risk industries operating in isolated areas that lacked a medical care infrastructure.[10] For example, mine operators and railroad companies hired company doctors to treat occupational accidents and to provide basic care to workers and their families (see chapter 2). These doctors were paid on a salary basis—a guaranteed income was often necessary to attract them to remote areas to care for low-wage workers—out of contributions deducted from workers' paychecks.

With the advent of state worker compensation laws in the second decade of the twentieth century, all employers were required to provide first-aid, medical, surgical, and hospital services for occupational injuries. By 1913, 21 states had such laws and by 1920, 43 states mandated employer coverage for accidents on the job.[11] While worker compensation laws did spark more employer interest in worker health care, this increase in attention was limited as employer liability was not always comprehensive. In fact, the laws tended to provide most relief in the form of cash benefits to compensate for lost income and provided little in terms of medical care. Funds for medical care commonly were capped and only available after a waiting period that hampered the ability of the worker to receive timely care.[12] For example, the laws did not require employers to pay for attending physician fees, the most expensive component of the health care bill.[13] Hence, employers' endeavors to minimize their liability exposure by improving the health of their workers were restricted to modest endeavors such as health examinations and plant engineering studies.[14]

Also in the early twentieth century, health plans emerged as welfare capitalism became fashionable among a small but prominent group of corporate leaders like Consolidated Edison, Endicott-Johnson, the Homestake Mining Company, and Standard Oil Company of Louisiana.[15] Adherents of welfare capitalism saw two potential gains from the provision of benefits like health care. First, the provision of health care would increase employee satisfaction and thereby heighten employee loyalty to the firm. Second, and related to the first reason, this increased worker satisfaction would also hinder unionization.

Employers failed to realize these advantages since they left employees to finance their own care. In this era, employers' involvement in health care typically was limited to administering commercial group policies that employees would purchase under plans called "mutual benefit associations."[16] Employers preferred this arrangement because they did not incur any risk and because it was less expensive than establishing a company-run plan. By leaving workers to foot the bill, however, employers realized little increase in employee loyalty.

Worker-financed commercial insurance policies had serious shortcomings which precluded their adoption beyond a small number of firms. The policies were limited to hospital and "nursing fees," and did not cover the charges of the attending physician. While supplementary medical care benefits could be purchased through life insurance plans, these policies often were prohibitively expensive for workers. Furthermore, policies typically were canceled when the policyholder reached age 60. As a result, by 1930 only 1.2 million employees (2 percent of the labor force) and an additional one to two million dependents were covered by commercial insurance policies.[17]

The eventual expansion of commercial group policies to include hospital, surgical, and medical indemnity coverage enabled employers to provide health benefits somewhat more successfully during the ascendance of the personnel management movement spawned by welfare capitalism. Here, the rationale for providing health benefits was augmented to include not only the enhancement of employee loyalty but also an increase in employee motivation and productivity. As such, employer plans became more comprehensive and, for the first time, employers began to provide care for alcoholism and mental illness.[18] In 1926, more than 400 companies operated their own plans, 92 percent of which had hospitals or emergency rooms and 63 percent of which were staffed by physicians.[19] A 1931 survey found

315 mutual benefit associations in operation, with an average age of 21 years of operation.[20]

Despite the fact that employers were often in a better financial position to provide the health benefits, their efforts only marginally outpaced those of the labor groups. To begin with, health benefits were expensive to provide, even for employers. More fundamentally, the extension of employer-sponsored plans was limited in the long term due to the dissatisfaction of workers and organized medicine. Discontent arose from the limited scope and duration of the plans, management's control over company physicians, and the potential for these plans to undercut physicians' incomes.

First, even at their prewar apex, workers viewed employer plans as too modest in their coverage. Despite the growing awareness of the importance of worker health, employers spent relatively little on health care. With the exception of employer-funded company doctor plans, most monies for health care were spent on physical examinations and plant engineering. A 1931 survey of employers sponsoring mutual benefit associations found that the most common criticism of the associations leveled by management itself was that benefits were inadequate and/or available for too short a period of time.[21] As was the case with their precursors, mutual benefit associations were more likely to provide sickness benefits than medical benefits, and as the 1931 survey noted, "Only a small fraction of the sick-benefit funds . . . at present are venturing into new fields; as a whole they are still essentially insurance organizations, making no attempt to control either the incidence or the severity of the illnesses afflicting their members."[22] The circumscribed nature of most employer plans limited their returns in terms of increased worker health and satisfaction.

In addition, workers still financed most of the costs of sickness and medical benefits. Over half of the respondents to the 1931 employer survey reported no contributions or only modest contributions to their employees' mutual benefit associations leaving the survey to conclude that employers more often engaged in "passive recognition" than in "active company support."[23] Furthermore, even at their height of development in the prewar period, employer plans were not on sound actuarial grounds with the result that many did not survive the normal cyclic economic downturns, much less the Depression. Since health benefits most commonly produce satisfaction over the long term, as employees have the need to avail themselves of medical attention, plans with short durations did not produce the returns to loyalty that employers expected.

Second, employers often were reluctant to develop health plans due to workers' dissatisfaction with company doctors. Workers argued that firms were interested simply in procuring the lowest bidder for the job with the result that company doctors had little incentive to provide high quality care. Furthermore, workers contended that the company doctor would ultimately hold management interests at heart. This was unacceptable to workers since, for instance, medical evaluation was key in determining awards in industrial injury claims. Organized labor, moreover, disliked the paternalistic nature of employer-provided health benefits.

Third, it is doubtful that organized medicine would have allowed a significant extension of contract medicine beyond geographically remote areas where a guaranteed salary was required to attract physicians. Organized medicine protested the practice of contract medicine outside of these areas and often prohibited its members from engaging in such an "exploitative" arrangement. The American Medical Association's (AMA) opposition to prepayment was aroused further when contract medicine was expanded to include the families of workers or other members of the community who otherwise would have paid for their care under more lucrative fee-for-service arrangements.[24]

Thus, even if management had devoted more resources to developing health plans, the long term viability of these plans was improbable. Labor resisted employer provision of health care because it usually was inadequate and it violated worker control of the choice of physician. Furthermore, organized medicine did not welcome contract medicine's infringement on physician autonomy and would have vigorously opposed the further expansion of contract medicine (see chapter 6). Without a developed system of third-party health insurance, management had little hope of overcoming the protests of both groups.

World War II and Employer Willingness to Bargain Over Health Benefits

World War II created conditions in the domestic economy that induced employers to bargain over health benefits. Employers were anxious to hide their excessive war profits from public scrutiny. They also were becoming increasingly concerned with the rise in shop floor militancy. The heightened volatility of labor was especially troublesome at a time when sustained production was necessary to meet wartime demand. As long as wartime price and wage freezes were in place, employers could not appease workers by increasing wages.

Management's interest in bargaining over health benefits was piqued when the War Labor Board ruled in 1942 that health programs that did not exceed five percent of payroll costs were acceptably noninflationary in the wartime economy. Employers noted that providing health benefits would both create an additional expense that would decrease unsightly profits, and also decrease workplace friction by increasing worker loyalty to the firm. Despite the fact that it was still not clear whether employers were required to bargain over health benefits under the Wagner Act,[25] many did not oppose labor's attempts to place this untested issue on the bargaining table. By 1945, the Bureau of Labor Statistics estimated that approximately 600,000 workers were covered by plans negotiated through collective bargaining. The number of covered workers doubled in the following two years to 1,250,000 and almost doubled again in the next year to reach a total of 3 million workers in 1947.[26]

Initially, however, despite the apparent willingness of employers to discuss health benefits, few unions were in the position to bargain for these benefits. Health plans were extraordinarily complicated benefits to establish and few unions had the resources and expertise necessary to engage in such costly negotiations. Moreover, the 1940s proved to be difficult bargaining terrain for labor. In the early war years most unions were preoccupied with the delicate balancing act of minimizing wildcat strikes while the no-strike pledge was in force and, at the same time, securing a portion of war profits for workers. After the war, strikes escalated and dampened public sympathy for labor. This growing disenchantment was evidenced by increasingly hostile public opinion and the passage of the Taft-Hartley Act. The inimical bargaining environment sapped labor of the energy necessary to bargain for health benefits.

Unions that could afford to bargain for fringe benefits found that it was relatively easier to raise public sympathy for health plans than for wage increases. Few could deny workers a remedy for injury and illness after they had exerted themselves heroically to meet the war demand. Elevated public consciousness over workers' lack of access to health care provided momentum for labor's drive for employer-provided health benefits.[27] In fact, the eventual attainment of health benefits would represent one of the few political victories for labor in the immediate postwar period.

The watershed event that secured the status of health benefits as a bargaining issue was the Supreme Court's 1948 Inland Steel decision which ruled that pensions could be considered a "condition of employment" under the Wagner Act. This decision confirmed for union and management negotiators that health plans also qualified as a bargaining issue under the Act. As a result, the number of workers covered by negotiated health plans increased from 2.8 million to 7 million in the two years following the Inland Steel ruling. Unions like those in the textile, apparel, and leather; lumber and furniture; trade, insurance, and finance; printing and publishing; and mining industries succeeded in bargaining for employer-financed health plans. These plans represented nearly 60 percent of all plans established through collective bargaining. Unions in the paper and allied products; petroleum, chemicals, and rubber; stone, glass, and clay; and metal products industries secured jointly-financed plans.[28] By 1960, 14.5 million union members and 22.6 million dependents, or 80 percent of the population covered under collective bargaining agreements, received coverage for hospitalization under their union contracts.[29]

Fundamentally, the cooperation of management and labor in the provision of health benefits illustrates a subtle but profound change in industrial relations underway in the immediate postwar period. In general, employers and union leaders expressed a desire to shift from a conflict management strategy to one of accommodation to better conform to the new bargaining landscape. Once the war demand slackened, fears of another depression were palpable and accommodation was seen as a more probable way of avoiding an economic downturn. Organized labor also had emerged from the 1930s and World War II as a force to be reckoned with; management could no longer afford to dismiss labor's demands. This was particularly true as employers in many sectors of American industry realized that they would need the help of labor leaders to implement productivity-enhancing technological change. A strategy of accommodation was more conducive to convincing union leaders to accept technological change which brought with it reductions in the workforce.

Types of Health Plans Adopted Through Collective Bargaining

Unions played a prominent role in the development of health care benefits during the postwar period. First, unions campaigned vigorously for the codification of health benefits as a staple in labor contracts. This effort resulted in widespread coverage of a sector of the population that previously had lacked access to the health care system. Unions also were successful in pressuring employers to expand the scope of benefits and to extend coverage to dependents and retirees. Second, unions expressed a prescient interest in the provision of cost-effective care long before employers or the state showed concern over cost escalation. Unions had strong incentives to contain costs as devoting more resources to health care detracted from advances in other areas of the collective bargaining agenda. As large purchasers of health care, unions were able to promote cost-containment measures that did not jeopardize quality in order to control costs.

Bargaining for health benefits involved not only deciding on which share of the costs employers and workers respectively would bear, but also deciding on the specific type of health coverage. Unions bargaining for benefits chose between two main avenues of health care delivery in the postwar period. Unions either established independent self-insured plans or they had employers purchase one of three types of commercial coverage: indemnity insurance, Blue Cross-Blue Shield insurance, or prepayment plans. Throughout the early years of negotiated health plans, self-insured plans like those of the UMWA and the ILGWU enjoyed the highest profile. However, most unions had neither the resources nor the member profile necessary to create and benefit from a self-insured plan. Consequently, the vast majority of unions elected coverage by commercial plans.

By 1960, 37 million workers and their dependents received hospitalization coverage—the most prevalent health benefit—as a result of collectively bargained plans. This group comprised 20.6 percent of the total U.S. population, 28.0 percent of the insured civilian population, and 79.9 percent of the population covered under collective bargaining agreements.[30] Table 1 shows that private insurance companies and Blue Cross-Blue Shield provided coverage for the vast majority of workers (a combined total of 89.1 percent) receiving benefits as a result of collective bargaining. Plans operated by unions or jointly by unions and employers covered only 2.7 million workers, or 7.3 percent of those workers covered under union contracts. Roughly 30 percent of these workers were beneficiaries of the UMWA's plan alone.

With the advent of negotiated employer-financing, a small vanguard of unions created independent, self-insured health plans in order to retain control over the provision of health care. Union leaders could derive increased rank-and-file allegiance to the union by directly administering a service that union members valued highly. In the case of the miners, by establishing an independent plan, the UMWA received virtually all of the credit for bringing modern health care to the coal fields even though coal operators financed the plan. However, with these tremendous gains also came a considerable risk of incurring political losses should the health plan falter. For instance, when the UMWA leadership decided to cut benefits and eligibility in an effort to shore up the Fund's sagging finances, rank-and-file protests

Table 1   Enrollment in collectively bargained health benefit plans, 1960

Type of Plan	Number Enrolled in millions (percentage distribution)			
	Hospital	Surgical	Medical	Major Medical
Insurance Companies	17.0 (45.9)	16.8 (46.7)	9.5 (38.0)	8.2 (74.5)
Blue Cross– Blue Shield	16.0 (43.2)	14.9 (41.4)	11.8 (47.2)	2.5 (22.7)
Union or Jointly Sponsored Plans	2.7 (7.3)	2.6 (7.2)	2.2 (8.8)	0.3 (2.7)
Other Plans	1.3 (3.5)	1.7 (4.7)	1.5 (6.0)	—
TOTAL	37.0	36.0	25.0	11.0

Source: U.S. Department of Health, Education, and Welfare, Public Health Service, Division of Community Health Services, *Health Economics Series* no. 1 "Medical Care Financing and Utilization," (Washington, D.C.: GPO, 1962): Table 85, 97.

were directed at the union's leadership. Because of the close association between the health plan and the union, few members thought to blame operators for insufficient contributions. Hence, the appealing political gains from administering independent plans were not immutable, but were subject to erosion and even reversal depending on the fortunes of the plan.

Even among the select group of unions that bargained for independent plans, the UMWA's plan would stand out as the most ambitious and exceptional. The most common independent plans established by unions took the form of union-run clinics.[31] At least initially, most clinics provided only diagnostic and ambulatory services, and only two unions provided comprehensive care through their clinics.[32] The Fund, by contrast, developed an extensive system of care, astutely integrating direct provision with savvy control over indirect provision of care.

With all the advantages of providing care directly to their members, why did not more unions establish independent plans? In practice, few unions were able to meet the prerequisites necessary to establish successful independent plans: a high volume of patients, minimal competition with existing patterns of medical care, and a considerable investment of resources. Only two major unions, the ILGWU and the UMWA, were positioned to develop the most significant and enduring independent plans. At the inception of their plans, both unions could provide the requisite volume of patients; both provided services that were otherwise unavailable and succeeded in providing the requisite financing for their plans. Moreover, the vision of the leaders of these unions was instrumental in providing a path-breaking system of health care for workers. Capitalizing on the strength of their unions, these leaders championed innovative and far-reaching solutions to address the enormous human cost that their industries extracted from the rank-and-file.

The broad contours of health plans available to miners always have differed markedly from the prevailing models of worker health care. Before World War II, in an era when few employers provided sustained access to quality medical care, mine operators commonly contracted company doctors to provide care throughout the fluctuations of the business cycle. The independent, union-controlled plan that the UMWA succeeded in negotiating after the war would again stand in striking contrast to typical third-party insurance plans most unions adopted.

The experience of the Fund presented in the following chapters must not be seen, then, as the standard pattern of health benefits enjoyed by union members and their families. Understanding the factors that allowed the Fund to diverge from the mainstream suggests some determinants of its accomplishments. It is equally important to understand, however, that in certain respects the conditions that the miners faced were not radically different from those that prevailed in other industries. Most notably, the conditions in the coal industry that allowed the UMWA to establish the Fund in the late 1940s (see chapter 2) were not significantly different from those that prevailed in other industrial sectors. This suggests that the pathbreaking nature of the Fund was not due solely to the unique attributes of the mining industry.

Finally, the innovative initiatives that Fund administrators sponsored that will be described in detail in later chapters should also be evaluated in light of efforts by other unions to increase the access to, quality of, and cost-effectiveness of care. Unions helped change the role of consumers in the health care field through their scrutiny of its delivery and financing mechanism. A number of influential unions demanded that providers be accountable to payers and, furthermore, that providers recognize that health care funds were bounded. Many unions promoted important health care reforms that identified the gains to be made from altering the incentives that providers face in prescribing and charging for treatment. Yet perhaps no union was better situated than the UMWA to initiate reforms in the delivery of care. The UMWA's ability to maximize its power as a direct payer and to marshal its resources to rationalize health care delivery stands virtually alone as an example of the full extension of the influence of organized labor into the health care arena.

Bargaining for Benefits: The Fund and the Transformation of Industrial Relations in the Coal Industry

*T*hroughout the late nineteenth and early twentieth centuries, miners had access to, at best, rudimentary health care. For a monthly fee, miners could expect a company doctor to care for everything from injuries suffered in mine accidents to the delivery of their children. Yet miners typically had no say in the choice of doctor the company employed and had little recourse if the company doctor was unacceptable. Moreover, miners found that the few hospitals available to them lacked adequate facilities.

In short, the quality of the health care available to the mining population matched their substandard housing stock, poor public sanitation, and inadequate means of transportation. Seen in this context, the accomplishments of the UMWA's Welfare and Retirement Fund in providing unparalleled medical care to a previously neglected group are even more striking. Within a decade, the union would succeed in replacing the company doctor system with a generously funded health plan which allowed miners, both retired and working, and their families to visit a range of physicians practicing in newly established clinics and hospitals. The level of care in the coalfields increased dramatically with the arrival of skilled medical professionals and the introduction of state-of-the-art medical technologies and procedures. When a beneficiary's condition required special attention, the Fund arranged for the patient to be transported to the best medical centers in the country.

Despite the fact that it was one of the first unions to fight for comprehensive health benefits, the UMWA's goals for their health plan were ambitious by both contemporary and current standards. Insisting on a reversal of the historical pattern of the provision of health benefits, the UMWA demanded that employers finance the benefits while the union assumed control of the Fund. The union spent five years working to realize this extraordinary arrangement. UMWA president John L. Lewis placed the demand for a comprehensive health plan on the bargaining table repeatedly throughout the second half of the 1940s; the rank-and-file struck to show that their determination to reform the pattern of care in the coalfields matched that of their leader.

A review of the period from 1945 to 1950 reveals that the evolution and fortunes of the coal industry itself had a considerable impact on the viability of the Fund. The health of the industry determined in large part the state of relations between the miners, their union, and the operators. This has affected the fate of the Fund from its inception. More specifically, the demand for coal and the rising competition from alternative fuels and from nonunion mines affected the bargaining positions of both the operators and the UMWA. Mutual recognition of this fact led to an agreement in 1950 that brought to an end the turmoil over the Fund and secured its existence. However, this agreement also determined that industry conditions would dictate the scope of the Fund.

Lewis's choice of a tonnage royalty system to provide funds for the health plan revealed how the fortunes of the Fund would be tied directly to the those of the industry. This system not only linked health funds to the production cycles in the coal industry, but also to the amount of coal that was produced by UMWA miners. The problems inherent in the tonnage royalty payment system would be revealed as it later became evident that the health needs of the covered population did not vary in proportion to the cycles of the industry nor to the prevalence of union-mined coal. Given the resulting disparity between the cost of beneficiary care and the monies provided by the tonnage royalty, by the late 1950s the Fund would experience shortfalls resulting in dire consequences for the operation and scope of the health plan.

This chapter relates the events at the negotiating table, at the mines, and in the industry that led to the creation of the Fund. Particular attention is given to the experiences and expectations of both management and labor that helped shape a new era of industrial relations in the coalfields. The new alliances that were formed during this time among the leaders of the coal industry would hinge critically on the Welfare and Retirement Fund.

Early Health Care Plans in the Coalfields

Physician Care: The Company Doctor

Until the creation of the Fund in the 1940s, company doctors were a standard feature of mining communities beginning as far back as the 1860s. The administration and provision of care by company doctors was fairly uniform throughout the coalfields. Company doctors were funded by monthly deductions from miners' paychecks collected by mine operators. In the early twentieth century, the monthly deductions were commonly set at 50 cents for single miners and one dollar for married miners.[1] This check-off entitled the miner and his dependents to unlimited office calls, house calls within a certain geographic area, and a limited range of basic pharmaceutical drugs and immunizations. Miners paid separate fees for services like the delivery of babies and the treatment of venereal diseases.

The check-off offered physicians fixed fee contracts for large populations and, as such, acted as a necessary incentive to attract doctors to remote mining towns. Physicians demanded that mining companies collect the health fees to avoid the high transactions costs of doing so themselves.[2] In essence, the check-off was a prepayment system—similar to that used by modern health maintenance organizations—that guaranteed physicians acceptable levels of income. By the late 1930s, the typical check-off rate had risen to $1.80 per month for married miners and $1.30 per month for single miners. Since, on average, 70 percent of miners were married, a small camp of 200 to 300 miners could "support a good doctor without difficulty" with an income of $3,960 to $5,940 annually.[3] The advantages offered by the prepayment system were so compelling that this feature of the check-off would survive the eventual demise of the company doctor system.

The most frequent criticism leveled at the company doctor system was the lack of choice the miners faced in obtaining care. Miners rarely had any say in the selection of the company doctor and seldom had access to other physicians. Miners had a variety of objections to operators' insistence upon choosing the company doctor. As a matter of principle, the miners and their union felt that the system was paternalistic. Miners argued that as long as they were paying for their care, they deserved the right to select the company physician.

As a matter of practice, miners complained that their inability to select and dismiss company doctors increased the likelihood that the doctors would be inaccessible, ill-trained, and/or biased in favor of the company. First, having a doctor who could provide timely care was critical given the unpredictable and often severe nature of mining accidents. Miners protested that since operators often hired doctors who had taken contracts with a number of communities, such doctors were usually overextended and thus less likely to be available in emergencies. There were numerous examples of company doctors caring for groups in excess of the national average level of patients. At a time when the national average was one doctor to 815 patients, a 1939 survey of medical care conditions in southern West Virginia found four doctors serving 15,000 patients (1 to 3,750); two doctors serving 5,000 patients (1 to 2,500); and three doctors serving 6,000 patients (1 to 2,000).[4]

Second, miners had limited recourse when they found the company doctor to be inadequately trained or otherwise lacking in the skills necessary to provide acceptable care. Company doctors typically were hired on the basis of whom they knew rather than how they were likely to perform. A government survey of medical care in the coalfields conducted in 1946 concluded that,

> physicians were not selected primarily on the basis of professional qualifications and the character of the facilities and services that were offered, but on the basis of personal friendships, financial tie-ups, social viewpoints, or other nonmedical considerations. Competition among doctors for prepayment contracts may be quite brisk. The quality of professional services that can be offered is a bargaining point, but it is known that doctors have occasionally obtained contracts by their talents for ingratiating themselves with company officials or leaders of the Union [the UMWA].[5]

Deprived of the right to hire and fire their doctors, miners were forced to tolerate substandard or even fraudulent care. For example, in one mining town the son of an elderly company doctor carried out his father's practice despite the fact that he had completed only one year of dental school.[6] District 29 (West Virginia) miners described the "chief medical benefits" from their physician check-off to be "a big red pill and an aspirin tablet."[7]

Third, miners protested that by retaining the right to hire and fire physicians, operators gained unwarranted control over the doctors' practices. As a result, company doctors were known to side with management in evaluations to determine workers' compensation,[8] to suspend their services during strikes, to perform physical examinations to find grounds to discharge miners active in the union, and even to serve as spies for the operators.[9] Lewis summarized,

> A company doctor does much more than treat the sick and injured. He acts as company representative in compensation cases. He is the company agent in insurance claims. He determines the physical fitness of job applicants. The company selects a doctor of its own choosing. Although his salary is paid out of deductions from the miners' wages, the doctor works for the company, not the employees. A doctor thus selected testifies against workers in compensation cases where the company disputes the extent of an employee's injuries. He does the company's bidding in passing upon the physical fitness of job applicants.[10]

A survey at seven West Virginia mines revealed that company doctors were four times less likely than "noncompany" doctors to submit industrial injury claims.[11] Not surprisingly, a common refrain heard throughout the coalfields was, "we would rather have a bad doctor we know we can trust than the best doctor in the world if he is controlled by the company."[12]

Miners were not only prevented from selecting their physicians, but they also were precluded from reviewing the financing of the system. A 1939 survey found that it was not uncommon for operators to hire physicians on salary and then keep the difference between the salary and the check-off payments received from the miners.[13] During hearings before the Senate Subcommittee of the Committee on Education and Labor in 1937, Senator Robert La Follette questioned a coal company official, Mr. Bassham, about the financing of the company's medical plan,

Sen. La Follette: You pay the doctors for the total medical services that they render $1,250 a month, and you take in from $1,800 to $2,400. Who gets the gravy?

Mr. Bassham: It goes to the company.[14]

Larger operators could realize substantial profits from administering the check-off system,

> Bethlehem Steel . . . had taken in a total of $31,215,571 and had spent $26,769,778. The steel corporation refused to render a detailed statement of expenditures. The surplus of $4,445,793 was at the disposal of the company, to invest as it saw fit. Three were no provisions . . . for liquidation or disbursement of the surplus among employees.[15]

In addition, some companies retained a 10 percent fee for collecting the check-off, a process that operators performed at little cost.[16]

Operators were not the only party to profit from the check-off system. The company doctors themselves often developed practices lucrative enough to vault them into mine ownership. A company doctor in Harlan county garnered enough income from check-off deductions from several mining communities that he was able to purchase and subsequently operate three mines. The UMWA district president for this area noted, "One cannot readily visualize this doctor testifying against himself in a compensation hearing."[17] Moreover, the check-off system created incentives for company doctors to reduce the quality of care they offered in order to maximize their earnings. As part of the Senate

Subcommittee hearings in 1937, Senator Elbert Thomas questioned
Bassham about these incentives,

> *Sen. Thomas:* You mentioned that the doctors pay for their own
> medical supplies out of the money you allot them . . .
> well, now, the more the doctor uses, then, the less he
> makes, doesn't he?
>
> *Mr. Bassham:* I think so; yes, sir.
>
> *Sen. Thomas:* What effect do you think that would have on a doctor?
>
> *Mr. Bassham:* Naturally, he would not use any more than is necessary.[18]

"Necessary," of course, was defined by the physician whose behavior was
unaffected by dissatisfaction on the part of patients who had no voice in his
selection or retention.

Miners who were dissatisfied with their company doctor had few opportunities to obtain care from other physicians. Only those miners who
resided close to metropolitan areas were sometimes able to receive care
from other physicians. However, since most basic health plans were com-
pulsory, miners who sought care elsewhere were forced to pay additional
fees for such care.[19] In at least one instance, miners resorted to striking in
order to remove a company doctor who had relayed covertly private opin-
ions expressed by patients to company officials.[20] Generally, however, miners found few effective ways of expressing discontent with company doctors
whom they found to be unacceptable. Hence, inadequate physician care
remained yet another facet of the miners' lamentable living conditions.

Hospital Care

The coalfields had a disproportionately large number of private hospitals
as compared to the national average. These hospitals allowed many miners
to purchase separate prepayment plans for hospital care as a supplement to
the care provided by their company doctor. Typically, hospitals themselves
offered the hospitalization plans although in a few cases, operators, local
unions, or nonprofit groups administered the hospitalization plans.
Hospitalization plans often were supported by check-off payments that the
company transferred directly to the hospitals. It was not unusual for the
operator or the company doctor to own the hospital, and for the company
doctor to be a stockholder in the mining operation, with the result that the
hospitals viewed "each case [as] a liability."[21]

The early history of these hospitalization plans is less complete than that of the company doctors. The few detailed accounts of miners' use of hospitals suggests that the hospital services available to miners and their families ranged from spartan infirmaries to relatively modern facilities. For instance, the Coxe family supported a number of the first miners' hospitals near their holdings in Hazelton, Pennsylvania, in the late nineteenth century. However, these hospitals often lacked the technology and staff to make them more than "a place for the dying."[22] By contrast, in 1911, doctors in Albia, Iowa, offered hospitalization coverage, including surgery, to miners and their families for only 50 cents a month. One of the doctors erected the hospital where covered miners received care, and he equipped it with "the latest modern equipment." This plan enjoyed the support of the local union leadership and was successful enough to be reproduced in Des Moines five years later.[23]

In general, however, it appears that only a small proportion of miners enjoyed access to hospitals. When the United States Coal Commission surveyed 167 coal towns in 1922, it found that while 147 of the towns (88 percent) had a resident physician, only 44 towns (26 percent) had hospitals. The study also noted the difficulties inherent in obtaining hospital care in remote areas,

> except for a few camps which had their own hospitals, the journey to the nearest hospital was often very difficult. In remote districts the roads were, for a large part, impassable. Train service was very limited. Unless special trains were made up, injured men might have to wait twelve hours or more and then have a train journey of six or eight hours.[24]

Thus, while miners who resided near urban areas were more likely to have access to hospitals outside of their communities, as a practical matter their ability to do so was dependent upon the availability of reliable means of transportation.

Hospitals that were accessible to miners were often crowded, resulting in long waits and unsanitary conditions. Patients commonly complained that they were rushed prematurely out of the hospital.[25] This situation was exacerbated by the penchant of hospitals to seek contracts, regardless of their capacity constraints.[26] For example, a 1939 survey found a 75-bed hospital which held contracts for 50,000 to 60,000 beneficiaries. Often hospitals engaged in such intense competition that rates were reduced to the point where services could not be provided adequately.[27]

While the record of miners' hospitalization experience is incomplete, the evidence that does exist suggests that few miners had access to quality hospital care. A UMWA official sent to research medical conditions in the coalfields noted during contract negotiations, "I want to say to you, as members of this [Bituminous Joint] conference, that in all my existence of 64 years I have never run into anything as vicious as the company doctors, the hospital set-up and the insurance. There is nothing in the U.S. like it that I have heard of, and in my opinion it has Al Capone skinned a city block."[28]

The Bureau of Cooperative Medicine found in its 1939 survey that this sentiment was also prevalent among the rank-and-file: "The miners interviewed, *without a single exception,* were dissatisfied with present medical conditions and hopeful that it would be possible to introduce some kind of change. A typical comment, frequently heard in all parts of the region, was: 'An improvement in medical conditions would mean more to us than a raise in pay.'"[29]

The Fund's Birth

Before the 1940s, despite its rudimentary nature, the miners' health care system was not a target for reform for two reasons. First, the care provided largely met the prevailing national standards at a time when patients generally were treated at home or in a doctor's office, and medical procedures and treatments were expected to cure only basic illnesses and injuries. Second, mining culture placed the onus of risk of illness and injury emanating from this dangerous profession primarily on the miner himself.[30] Miners reluctantly accepted the risk of death from mine accidents and endured illnesses caused or aggravated by conditions in the mines without expecting much aid from the state or from their employers. It was the miners themselves, and not the physicians or hospitals that treated them, who were considered to be ultimately responsible for mining's effect on their health.

By the 1940s, however, changes in medicine and in the standing of miners rendered these explanations obsolete and, consequently, brought critical attention to the state of health care in the coalfields. First, the pace of medical advances had increased dramatically in the interwar years and the contributions of science to the war effort gave unprecedented support to the rapid diffusion of innovations in medical treatments and technologies.[31] As this progress bypassed mining towns, the gap between the health of residents of mining communities and that of the general population widened noticeably.

Second, the UMWA found itself in a better position to question the validity of the assumption that its members bore mining's consequences to their health. The strength and prominence of the UMWA was perhaps at its peak during the 1940s as a result of a decade's worth of organizing drives and coal's importance as a supplier for basic industries in the wartime economy. As a result, John L. Lewis received public attention when he used contract negotiations as a bully pulpit to decry the industry's practice of replacing instead of rehabilitating injured workers. This increased the pressure on operators to accede to the demands of a workforce that was organized to protest inferior pay, benefits, and working conditions.

The newly empowered miners channeled their frustrations over inadequate health care into a demand for employer-financed health benefits on an industry-wide scale. This unprecedented demand required the operators to make an investment of funds and a long-term commitment to their workers on a scale that challenged the entire structure of relations within the industry. Under ordinary circumstances, mine owners could have been expected to reject Lewis's health care proposals outright. However, the war and the immediate postwar reconversion period brought two critical developments that forced the operators to bargain over health benefits: the boom in demand for coal and the federal government's sanctioning of bargaining for benefits.

The coal industry as a whole was in better shape economically than ever before to provide health benefits. Enjoying huge wartime profits, mine owners could not claim that they lacked funds to provide health benefits to the workers whose efforts had helped generate those profits. Furthermore, the immediate postwar years did not bring a downturn in the industry as shown in Tables 2 and 3. Instead, the nation continued its heavy dependence on coal to fuel the postwar industrial boom. In 1945 coal comprised half of U.S. energy consumption. Coal production reached an all-time high in 1947, and while production fell slightly in 1948, it remained at wartime levels. Exports also reached new heights as European producers reconstructing from the war were unable to fuel Europe's recovery. Once wartime price controls were lifted, coal prices surpassed even the high levels posted after the First World War. Finally, coal's profitability, as measured by its after-tax return on investment, actually increased after the war. The industry registered a striking 9.5 percent return on investment in 1947 and 1948, tripling the returns of the previous two years.[32]

With the industry in a position to fund health benefits, the event that triggered negotiations on employer-financed health benefits came in 1942 when the War Labor Board ruled that health programs that did not exceed five percent of payroll costs were acceptable in the wartime economy.

Table 2 Coal Consumption, million tons, 1945–1960

Year	Domestic Consumption						Exports	Coal as % of Energy
	Utility	Steel	Rail	Retail	Other	Total		
1945	72	110	125	119	134	560	28	50.7%
1946	69	95	110	99	127	500	41	47.5
1947	86	119	109	97	135	546	69	47.2
1948	96	121	95	87	121	520	46	42.9
1949	81	102	68	89	106	446	28	39.9
1950	83	115	61	84	111	454	25	37.8
1951	102	125	54	74	114	469	57	35.8
1952	103	107	38	67	104	419	48	32.4
1953	112	122	28	60	105	427	34	31.6
1954	115	92	17	52	87	363	31	28.1
1955	141	115	15	53	99	423	51	29.3
1956	155	113	12	49	104	433	69	28.4
1957	157	115	8	36	98	414	76	27.1
1958	153	84	4	36	90	367	50	24.3
1959	166	86	3	29	82	366	37	23.1
1960	174	88	2	30	86	380	37	23.2

Sources: U.S. Department of Interior, Bureau of Mines, *Minerals Yearbook* (1965), 50. Peter Navarro, "Union Bargaining Power in the Coal Industry, 1945–1981," *Industrial and Labor Relations Review* 26, (January 1983): 227–28.

Table 3 Coal production, 1890–1952

Year	Tons (millions)	Average Price	Average Price[a] (1940)	Mines	Miners[b] (thousands)	Average Number of Days Worked Per Year
1890	111.3	$0.99			192	226
1895	135.1	$0.86		2,555	240	194
1900	212.3	$1.04			304	234
1905	315.1	$1.06		5,060	461	211
1910	417.1	$1.12		5,818	555	217
1915	442.6	$1.13		5,502	557	203
1920	568.7	$3.75		8,921	640	220
1925	520.1	$2.04		7,144	588	195
1930	467.5	$1.70		5,891	493	187
1935	372.4	$1.77		6,315	462	179
1940	460.8	$1.91	$1.91	6,324	439	202
1941	514.1	$2.19	$1.97	6,822	457	216
1942	582.7	$2.36	$1.88	6,972	462	246
1943	590.2	$2.69	$2.05	6,620	416	264
1944	619.6	$2.92	$2.21	6,928	393	278
1945	577.6	$3.06	$2.27	7,033	383	261
1946	533.9	$3.44	$2.24	7,333	396	214
1947	630.6	$4.16	$2.20	8,700	419	234
1948	599.5	$4.99	$2.44	9,079	442	217
1949	437.9	$4.88	$2.51	8,559	434	157
1950	516.3	$4.84	$2.40	9,429	416	183
1951	533.7	$4.92	$2.19	8,009	373	203
1952	466.8	$4.90	$2.24	7,275	335	186

[a]Real coal prices (1940) are computed using the wholesale price indices reported in the Bureau of the Census, *Statistical Abstract of the United States*.

[b]From 1890 to 1945, "Miners" reports the actual number of miners employed. From 1946 to 1952, "Miners" measures the average number of miners working daily.

Source: U.S. Department of the Interior, Bureau of Mines, *Minerals Yearbook* (1965), 50–51.

Deducting the expense of providing health benefits thus enabled operators to reduce the excessive wartime profits they were anxious to shield
from public scrutiny. Moreover, bargaining for health benefits filled the
void in negotiations created by the price and wage freezes. Operators concerned with maintaining production during the boom could offer health
benefits in lieu of wage increases to meet workers' demands and keep
operations running without disruption.

Yet state sanctioning of bargaining for benefits and favorable industry
conditions did not make operators' acceptance of health plans a foregone
conclusion. The lengthy negotiations that led to the establishment of the
Fund were marked not only by bargaining over the amount and nature of the
operators' monetary contributions but, more fundamentally, by disputes
over which side ultimately would dictate the terms of the agreement. In addition, both the operators and the union were forced to confront the changing
fortunes of the industry, the intervention of the federal government, and the
shifting sympathies of the public as they fashioned a compromise. The compromise they achieved in the 1950s would cement a new era of industrial
relations in coal and secure the future of the Fund.

The 1945 Contract Negotiations

John L. Lewis first raised the demand for an employer-financed, union-run
health and welfare fund during contract negotiations in 1945.[33] Employing
the business rhetoric of the operators, Lewis remarked, "the cost of caring for
the human equity in the coal industry is inherently as valid as the cost of
replacement of mining machinery, or the cost of paying taxes, or the cost of
paying interest indebtedness or any other factor incident to the production of
a ton of coal for the consumers' bins."[34] While robust industry conditions and
the War Labor Board's ruling forced them to listen to Lewis's proposal, operators initially showed little interest in making this concession. Operators proffered a variety of reasons for their opposition to providing health benefits:
they were unconvinced that the provision of health benefits would ensure
peaceful labor relations; they were anxious about the scope of the financial
commitment required; and they feared the industry could potentially revert
to its previously depressed state once the war and reconversion ended.

The operators received support from both the public and the government
in their opposition to the establishment of an employer-financed health plan.
The public had little experience with employer-financed, union-controlled
plans of the scope suggested by Lewis. In 1945 the Department of Labor

examined the 12,000 collective bargaining agreements in its files and found that only 600,000 workers were covered by health plans created through collective bargaining.[35] This number represented only 1 percent of the civilian workforce and reflected conditions in a only handful of industries. Moreover, the scope of medical care provided by most of these negotiated plans was limited to fixed rate payments for hospital care and surgery.

In addition, the public was unlikely to be persuaded by the union's arguments given their growing impatience with organized labor's expanding role in the national economy. The middle and upper classes aligned themselves with management out of weariness engendered by the postwar wave of strikes and fear that labor's demands were becoming boundless. This suspicion of labor's motives was fueled by the media's characterization of Lewis's health crusade as a transparent ploy to win the public support that had not materialized when the union's demands had been focused on more purely economic issues.[36]

With the exception of the War Labor Board's ruling, the state also largely sided with management against the UMWA's demand for a health plan. Specifically, Labor Secretary Frances Perkins rejected the union's plan during her participation in the 1945 negotiations. More broadly, the postwar years were characterized by a steady erosion of the gains the state had granted labor in the 1930s. Congress's passage of the Taft-Hartley Act in 1947 would represent the culmination of the increasing limitations on labor promulgated during the war, and would effectively end unfettered use of Wagner Act. Some legislators went so far as to attempt to outlaw employer-financed health, welfare and retirement funds outright.[37]

In the end, with the aid of public support, the operators successfully derailed Lewis's campaign for health benefits. Moreover, the fact that the contract negotiated in 1945 did not contain Lewis's health care proposal was not only an indication of the strength of operator opposition but also an indication of Lewis's as yet irresolute commitment to the demand. The 1945 negotiations demonstrated that attainment of an unprecedented demand of such a sizable scale required a concerted effort on the part of the union both to convince the public that Lewis's health plan was a reasonable and necessary demand, and to convince the operators that the industry would not function without it.

The 1946 Contract Negotiations

The next year John L. Lewis opened contract negotiations with the demand for a health plan at the top of the union's agenda. This time Lewis launched a more concerted and aggressive drive to increase public support for a new health plan for miners. In addition, in 1946 the union was prepared to disrupt the industry in order to convince the operators that health benefits were a priority for miners. The union's increased commitment to the demand for health was matched by equally ardent opposition from the operators. The turbulent year that it took to reach an agreement was marked by a remarkable chain of events—strikes, an injunction, fines, and an unprecedented exercise of state control over the industry.

Lewis first pitched his campaign for health benefits to the miners themselves. Miners needed little convincing that their access to medical care was inadequate. However, Lewis presented a vision for change and argued that better conditions could be won through collective bargaining. Rejecting the accepted wisdom in the industry that miners were responsible for their own well-being, Lewis contended that the operators were responsible for the health of their workers. If operators were required to tend to their machines, Lewis argued, surely it was logical that they afford their workers the same "upkeep."

The demand for health benefits was much more extensive than one for increased wages and, therefore, could not be achieved simply by sacrificing wage increases.[38] Miners would have to be mobilized to fight for health care for themselves and their families. In the spring of 1946, the pages of the *United Mine Workers Journal* reinforced the need for an overhaul of the miners' medical care system by highlighting a series of personal stories of health and safety tragedies. The two April issues featured cover photos of an orphaned child and of a disabled miner and his family, both carrying the caption "One Reason for a Welfare and Retirement Fund." The plights of miners and their families were collected and related in stories like "Affidavits Reveal the Tragic Story of Inadequate Compensation for Miners," and "'It's About Time We Got a Break,' says Injured Miner Who Can't Get Medical Care."[39] The latter story featured the predicament of Walter Shank, a 35-year union member who had been paralyzed from the waist down as a result of a 1943 mining accident. He had been released from the hospital when state compensation funds ran out after two years and, once home, found that his $16 monthly disability allotment was insufficient to maintain his family and pay for the medical care he required. Frustrated by his situation, Shank noted: "Our government is spending millions on foreign relief. While we miners gave all that we had to produce the coal that our country needed to win the war, now we can't get enough for food and medical care we need to relieve our suffering."[40] Stories like these rallied the miners around the demand for a health plan and create the rank-and-file commitment necessary for Lewis to bargain successfully for health benefits.

Repeatedly during the negotiations, Lewis eloquently and forcefully argued that the union would not settle without an employer-financed, union-run health plan. The operators largely ignored Lewis's oration, despite its increased intensity, and seemed prepared to sit through Lewis's performance just as they had in the previous year. After a month of fruitless negotiations, Lewis decided that the time had come to show the operators that the depth of the union's commitment to the health plan went beyond heightened rhetoric. On April 1, 340,000 miners backed up Lewis by walking out of the mines.

During the postwar boom in the demand for coal, the union possessed formidable ability to disrupt the industry. Coal reserves burned down to dangerously low levels and within weeks the depletion threatened to close plants. The steel industry cut its production in half and the auto industry shut down completely. The Office of Defense Transportation severely limited both freight and passenger rail service.[41]

The danger to the national economy posed by the interruption in the flow of its major energy sources prompted the government to get directly involved in bringing order to the industry. Initially, the state's participation worked to Lewis's advantage for three reasons. First, the government appeared to be more anxious than the operators to halt the depletion of the nation's coal reserves and restore the supply of energy to the rest of the economy. As a result, the government swiftly secured the operators' agreement "in principle" to the creation of the health plan. This concession allowed Lewis to order the miners back to work.

Second, the government's involvement in the negotiations reduced the operators' ability to renege on agreements. Shortly after the miners returned to the pits, the operators quickly distanced themselves from their stated commitment to the health plan. Angered by this turn of events, President Harry Truman ordered Secretary of the Interior Julius A. Krug to seize the mines and negotiate with the union. The operators were left on the sidelines as Lewis and Krug sat down for talks intended to secure the future of the Fund.

Third, the government proved to be vastly more sympathetic than the operators to the miners' plight. Krug himself met with health policy experts and became convinced of the validity of miners' demands for improved health care. This persuaded him to sign an accord with Lewis on May 29, 1946, that met the union's demands and ended the strike. The Krug-Lewis Accord included a health plan to be jointly supervised by the UMWA and the government. In addition, the accord authorized a government survey of medical conditions in the coalfields. Originally, the purpose of the survey was the seemingly uncontroversial task of discovering whether Lewis's allegations of widespread neglect could be substantiated. However, its publication a year later would play a pivotal role in compelling the operators and the union to reach an agreement similar to the Krug-Lewis agreement.

Initially, state intervention helped further the union's aims by creating the conditions needed for serious negotiations over the health plan. It soon became clear, however, that all three parties had different expectations for the implementation of the Krug-Lewis Accord. The operators felt little pressure to implement features of an agreement that was negotiated without their participation. Krug was noticeably lax in pushing the state into action once the crisis had been dealt with. Finally, Lewis became increasingly angered by the inaction of both the operators and Krug. Thus, barely four months after the accord was reached, Lewis registered his protest by calling for new contract negotiations with Krug. In addition, Lewis set a November 15 strike deadline in order to spur the operators and the federal government into action.

Lewis's bold move soured his relations with Krug. The union now replaced the operators as the party which endangered labor relations in the industry through actions that were viewed as irresponsible. Little progress was made in the talks that followed. Lewis stubbornly held to his position and, ignoring an injunction, lead the miners out of the pits on November 15. The strike served to increase the wrath of the federal government and, in December, the UMWA and Lewis were fined for contempt of court. Given these circumstances, the potential for productive discussions appeared dim and prolonging the strike seemed destined only to produce more fines. Sensing imminent defeat, Lewis ordered the miners back to work.

The spectacle of huge personalities wrestling for control of the bargaining process had caused attention to drift away from the substance of the negotiations. It took a major mining disaster to refocus concern on the miners' need for immediate improvements in safety and health conditions. In March 1947, a mine blast in Centralia, Illinois took the lives of 111 miners. Since the mines were still under Secretary Krug's control, Lewis used the disaster both to embarrass the government and to highlight the need for adequate health and safety measures.

The Centralia mine had been inspected twice in the previous six months and found in violation of the Federal Mine Safety Code on both occasions. The second inspection had occurred just five days before the tragedy and had revealed violations of the type that could lead to explosions. However, ignoring provisions of the Krug-Lewis Accord, the Centralia operators neither moved the miners nor closed the pits.[42] The disaster received so much public attention that in April the House of Representatives convened a subcommittee to investigate the incident. This gave Lewis a public forum in which to testify about Krug's neglect in enforcing provisions of the Krug-Lewis Accord.[43]

The Centralia disaster served to turn attention back to the substance of the negotiations. The explosion was shortly followed by the publication of the medical survey mandated by the Krug-Lewis Accord. This survey would indicate that the health and safety conditions that had produced the events at Centralia were not isolated occurrences but, rather, symptomatic of the substandard level of attention given to the health and safety of miners.

The Boone Report

As part of the Krug-Lewis agreement in 1946, the government agreed to sponsor a comprehensive survey of the health care available to miners and their families. Rear Admiral Joel T. Boone of the Navy's Medical Corps, a respected impartial observer, supervised a team from the Navy that evaluated conditions in coalfields from Pennsylvania to Washington during the summer of 1946. A year later, the team issued their results in *A Medical Survey of the Bituminous-Coal Industry,* better known as the "Boone Report."

This exhaustive survey of 260 mines employing roughly 72,000 miners detailed the availability and quality of health care offered to miners and their families.[44] As shown in Table 4, 60 percent of mines employing 73 percent of the miners surveyed contracted company doctors, and 66 percent of mines provided prepaid hospitalization plans. At 27 percent of the mines, neither plan was available.[45] It should be noted that the report's findings were based on mines producing more than 50,000 tons of coal per year so that the resulting depiction of the industry's health care system is probably not representative of the conditions at smaller mines.[46]

The report cited three major flaws in the delivery of physician and hospital care in the coalfields: the lack of choice of physician, the limited scope of coverage provided under health plans, and the substandard quality of facilities. First, the report supported the miners' contention that their inability to choose their own doctors adversely affected the quality of care they received. As noted previously, this system engendered abuses that typically resulted in the hiring of poorly qualified or otherwise unacceptable physicians. The

Table 4 Distribution of mines with prepayment plans for basic medical
care (company doctor check–off plans) and hospitalization, 1946

| Area | Number of Miners Surveyed | Number of Miners | Basic Check–off | | Hospital Plan (% of Mines) |
			% of Miners	% of Mines	
N. Appalachia	92	25,220	66%	47%	45%
S. Appalachia	107	35,007	93	86	96
Midwest	32	7,748	0	0	28
Plains	9	870	34	33	56
West	20	3,011	95	85	70
TOTAL	260	71,856	73%	60%	66%

Source: U.S. Coal Mines Administration, *A Medical Survey of the Bituminous–Coal Industry* (Washington, 1947), 119, 138–139.

report also included a variety of other illustrations of management's abuse of its control over company doctors. For example, the survey team uncovered instances where doctors were hired by the company on the condition that they perform pre-employment physicals and treat industrial injuries at no charge to the company. Since workers' compensation laws deemed these procedures to be the responsibility of the employers, the report concurred with miners' claims that they unjustly subsidized this care.[47]

The report also charged hospitalization plans with restricting miners' choice of hospitals and physicians to the detriment of the quality of care provided:

> Inherent within the system are opportunities for stifling competition and for establishing or entrenching monopolistic control of hospital service and of hospital and medical practice. The commanding position attained by a single hospital . . . or by a few physicians through the handling of all or nearly all of the contract practice in a given area, minimizes the professional opportunities of others to enter the area on a free competitive basis with any assurance of reasonable income. Thus the objectives of progressive medicine are defeated. The lack of competitive pressure in certain coal-mining communities permits substandard service to be supplied and dulls the incentives for improving medical service.[48]

This result was particularly unfortunate given that hospitals otherwise had the potential to attract physicians, especially sorely needed specialists, to underserved areas. However, as long as hospitals were forced to rely solely upon capitation payments, the incentive to restrict entry and reduce the scope of care provided remained powerful.

Second, the report found the range of services provided under the typical company doctor and hospitalization contracts to be inadequate in a number of ways. For example, the report leveled blunt criticism of the standard exclusion of treatment for venereal disease and obstetrical care from both the physician and hospitalization plans. As a result, beneficiaries often abstained from seeking treatment in order to avoid paying extra charges. Venereal disease, therefore, was quite pervasive in the coalfields despite the fact that contemporary advancements in the use of antibiotics could have eradicated it. Substantial reductions in high infant and maternal mortality rates could also have been achieved by removing the financial barriers to providing proper pre- and postnatal care, physician-assisted births, and hospital deliveries.[49]

Moreover, the report charged that the health plans available to miners and their families rarely provided satisfactory access to specialist care. The basic check-off plans did not provide specialist care since company doctors were, almost without exception, general practitioners. Hospitalization plans were more likely to provide specialist care, especially since the majority of these plans included coverage for surgical procedures. However, the report found that hospitalization plans typically included ambiguous language when it came to providing care beyond the most basic services. Hospitalization plans usually defined their scope according to "so-called understandings and common agreements," which often restricted the range of services that the plan included without charge.[50] Thus even when, in theory, access to specialist care appeared to be available as part of a hospitalization plan, in practice, many miners found these services required additional payments that they could not afford.

Third, the report revealed that most miners received care in substandard facilities. For instance, the survey team found that less than seven percent of the mines had "erected and equipped excellent dispensaries which are utilized for industrial medicine and ordinary medical care of miners and their dependents."[51] Most company doctors saw their patients in offices which ranged from "unattractive" to "insanitary."[52] Furthermore, the report found fully three-quarters of the hospitals surveyed to be deficient in at least one of the following basic facilities: surgical rooms, delivery rooms, labor rooms and nurseries, clinical laboratories, and X-ray facilities.[53]

Thus the Boone Report presented ample evidence to support miners' claims that health care conditions in mining communities were in desperate need of improvement. It concluded: "The present practices of medicine in the coal fields on a contract basis cannot be supported. They are synonymous with many abuses. They are undesirable and, in numbers of instances, deplorable."[54] The report rejected the operators' claims that weak or unstable financial conditions at the mines were the cause of inadequate medical care. In fact, the report concluded that the industry was perfectly capable of providing reasonably priced, high quality health care within the basic framework of the widespread prepayment plans.

The Boone Report served to raise public consciousness about the miners' dire living conditions. It unequivocally affirmed Lewis's claims that change was needed, and even suggested that the union assume an expanded role in the administration of a new industry-wide health plan. Together the Boone Report and the Centralia disaster had provided the union's demand for a health plan with legitimacy and a sense of urgency. As a result, the operators could no longer summarily dismiss the union's proposal for a new health plan for the miners.

The 1947 and 1948 Negotiations

By the spring of 1947, after a year of turmoil, the bargaining process had come full circle. Once again, the UMWA's demand for a health plan received attention and sympathy, this time extending beyond Krug to include the general public. Once again, industry conditions hastened the need for an agreement.

Collective bargaining between the union and the operators resumed after the government's authority to manage the mines expired in June. The negotiations were infused with a new spirit as a result of the desire of both sides to reach an agreement. Operators were eager to protect the sizable profits emerging from what was shaping up to be one of coal's best years. Lewis hoped to capitalize on growing public sentiment for the health plan during a time when operators would have funds available for the plan. In addition, Lewis cast a wary eye at the deliberations over the Taft-Hartley Act in progress in Washington. Having experienced everything government intervention had to offer, Lewis wanted to prove that private collective bargaining was a superior form of dispute resolution.[55]

The new tenor of talks speeded the pace of the negotiations and an agreement was signed by the operators and the UMWA in July. Containing most of the elements of the Krug-Lewis Accord, the contract's most prominent feature was the creation of a Welfare and Retirement Fund to provide health benefits, pensions, and widows' and survivors' benefits. The Fund transferred the cost of health care to the operators and the control of the provision of care to the union. The Fund would be administered without the government participation stipulated in the Krug-Lewis Accord. Instead, the Fund would be run by what was to become a more common arrangement in American labor relations: a tripartite trusteeship with one trustee to be chosen by the union, one by the operators, and the third neutral trustee to be chosen jointly by the other two members.[56] The trustees were given a broad statement of purpose and were left to determine eligibility, the scope of benefits, and investment strategies. The Fund would be financed by a royalty—initially set at 5 cents per ton—assessed on the amount of coal produced by union mines.

The establishment of the Fund was a extraordinary achievement for the UMWA. The 1947 contract promised miners a new system of comprehensive, modern care to replace the outdated, inadequate check-off plans. Illnesses and injuries sustained in the most dangerous of professions now would be met with quality treatment and rehabilitation instead of misery and death. However, it soon became apparent that instead of ending the conflict over the Fund, the contract simply shifted the battle lines; the Fund was now a reality, but its scope was still open for debate.

The operators crafted an extensive plan of attack on the Fund which unleashed three more years of confrontation and at several points threatened the Fund's very existence. Initially, the operators allowed Lewis to dictate the scope of plan in order to preserve the industry's fragile peace during a time of high profits. Concurrently, however, the operators instructed their trustee, Ezra Van Horn, to debilitate the Fund in any way possible.[57] Van Horn's actions would throw the Fund into another year-long crisis.

Van Horn met with the Fund's other two trustees, Lewis and neutral trustee Thomas Murray, throughout the summer and fall of 1947.[58] While Lewis and Murray offered proposals, Van Horn never suggested a proposal from the operators' side. Van Horn proved to be so intransigent that negotiations over the shape of the Fund stalemated to the point that Murray resigned in frustration.[59] The impasse deepened as both Lewis and Van Horn realized that they would never agree on another neutral trustee now that the operators' objectives had been revealed. Lewis's patience with the operators' thinly veiled desire to dismantle the Fund wore thin after eight months of negotiations with Van Horn. In March 1948, Lewis described to UMWA members, in no uncertain terms, the progress of the talks. He charged the operators and their trustee with "dishonoring" and "defaulting" on the Fund. His words had their intended effect: an "unofficial" six-week walkout of more than 200,000 miners began. Once again, the courts fined the union and Lewis for contempt and President Truman was given the opportunity to invoke an 80-day injunction now available under the Taft-Hartley Act.

The pattern of events in the spring of 1948 was strikingly similar to the events of late 1946. Once again the state intervened in an attempt to bring the two sides together. The first step was to find a replacement for Murray. Styles Bridges, a Republican senator from New Hampshire was accepted by both Lewis and Van Horn to be the neutral trustee. Bridges would side with Lewis consistently during the first year and a half of his tenure. Most notably, in the spring of 1948, Lewis and Bridges voted to activate the Fund, naming Lewis as its administrator and his confidante Josephine Roche as its director. This voting record prompted Van Horn to file a suit against both Lewis and Bridges that argued that the trustees' decisions be passed by unanimous and not majority vote.

While the deadlock in the Fund's negotiations had been ended, the new round of contract talks that began in May 1948 appeared to be headed for breakdown. As both sides prepared themselves for the inevitable extension of conflict from the bargaining table to the mines, the courts unexpectedly dismissed Van Horn's suit against Lewis and Bridges. Upholding the right of the trustees to enact decisions based on majority votes, the decision undermined the operators' attempt to subvert the Fund. Van Horn's strategy had backfired at a critical juncture. Within two days, the operators abandoned their efforts to destroy the Fund from within and agreed to a new contract which doubled its funding.

The Industry Downturn and the Threat to the Fund

The coal industry enjoyed a respite from labor-management conflict in the year following the 1948 contract. It had been more than three years since Lewis had first raised the proposal for the Fund and it finally seemed that the union's energy could be turned to the practicalities of improving its members' access to quality health care. During the summer of 1948, Roche appointed the Fund's administrative staff, and together they began designing the Fund's structure. John L. Lewis proudly handed out the Fund's first pension check in September.

By the time contract negotiations opened in the spring of 1949, however, the operators were ready to launch a final attempt to destroy the Fund. The first quarter results in 1949 signaled the possible end to the boom in demand for coal.[60] This downturn in demand combined with the weakening competitive position of union mines lead the operators to forecast correctly that the era of high profits was coming to an end. By the end of the year, production would have fallen back to prewar levels of output and prices would have leveled off.

There were three structural shifts underway in the energy market that contributed to the decrease in the demand for union coal: competition from alternative fuels, European producers' recovery from the war, and the growth of small, nonunion mines. First, increased competition from oil and gas posed the most significant threat to coal's dominance as an energy source for the U.S. economy. After the war, domestic oil fields expanded and oil fields in the Middle East were developed. As the expansion of supplies drove down prices, homes and businesses began switching to oil and gas. By the late 1940s switching became perceptible as plants completed the capital investments needed to use alternative fuels, railroads replaced coal-burning steam locomotives with diesel engines, and homeowners switched to cleaner and cheaper fuels. As a result, consumption of coal declined in both absolute and relative terms. From 1945 to 1949, domestic coal consumption decreased from 560 million tons to 446 million tons, and coal as a percentage of all energy consumed in the United States decreased from 50.7 percent to 39.9 percent (see Table 2).

Second, by 1949, as European producers showed signs of recovery from the war, Europe began reducing its dependence on U.S. coal imports. After the war U.S. exports had skyrocketed to 41 million tons in 1946, 69 million tons in 1947, and 46 million tons in 1948 (see Table 2). By 1949, once the European coal industry completed its recovery, exports slipped back to 28 million tons.

Third, eyeing the buoyant demand for coal, small mines capitalized on the relatively low barriers to entry in the coal industry and threatened the market share of the large, union operators. These nonunion mines saw their presence grow as the number of mines swelled from less than 7,000 mines during the war to between 8,000 to 9,000 in the immediate postwar period (see Table 3). The practices of the Tennessee Valley Authority (TVA), a major coal consumer in a region of the country known for its antipathy toward organized labor, also aided the growth of small, nonunion mines.[61] Created to promote industrial development in Appalachia by providing consumers with inexpensive fuel, the TVA's purchasing policies did little to support the formation of markets that would benefit union operators or miners. By awarding contracts to the lowest bidder, regardless of the mine's amount of production, wages, or benefits, the TVA fostered the growth of small, nonunion mines. These mines could win TVA contracts since they enjoyed lower production costs. Their nonunion status allowed them to pay lower wages and avoid making royalty payments to the Fund. In addition, mines employing fewer than 16 workers were exempt from federal safety laws and the concomitant considerable investment in capital and alternative production practices that often hampered productivity.

Union operators watched competition from alternative energy sources, European producers, and small mines erode their profits. As in the past, operators targeted labor costs as a way to cut costs and remain profitable. Specifically, the operators began watching closely the drain on revenues caused by their contributions to the Fund. When contract negotiations opened in May 1949, just as the downturn in the industry became perceptible, both Lewis and the operators came to the table sensing that the Fund would once again assume a central role in the talks. Once the contract expired on June 30, the operators wasted no time in voicing their desire to reduce their financial obligations to the Fund. The southern operators immediately suspended their payments to the Fund. In response, Lewis placed union miners on a three-day work week and watched the Fund's coffers drain. By the fall, the Fund skirted insolvency, prompting Lewis and Bridges to vote to stop paying benefits.[62]

The fall of 1949 witnessed a repeat of the events of the spring of 1948. Lewis informed the UMWA membership of the operators' latest ploy to dismantle the Fund, prompting a two- month work stoppage to protest the cessation of payments by the operators and the subsequent suspension of disbursements by the Fund. Rank-and-file discontent was deeper than in 1948 since miners resented having to fight again for a concession they thought they had already won. Miners also had begun to enjoy the benefits of the Fund's operations and were eager to protect their new health plan. The miners' resolve to safeguard the Fund revived the fall work stoppage after a brief hiatus in December in the form of a series of wildcat strikes in January and February of 1950.

With the industry in chaos and both sides retreating into irreconcilable positions, the federal government once again intervened in search of a solution. President Truman assumed a public role in the conflict in an effort to end four years of struggle in the coalfields. In November 1949, Truman announced that he was willing to invoke a Taft-Hartley injunction if reserves fell to emergency levels. Plagued by the wildcat strikes that followed in the months after Truman's announcement, the operators searched for a way to prod Truman into enjoining the strikes. In February, northern and captive mine[63] operators joined the southern operators in their suspension of payments to the Fund. The operators' actions had the desired effect of turning the wildcat strikes into a nationwide strike, prompting the courts to order the miners back to work and the union back to the table. This time, however, Lewis's appeal to workers to return to work was defied.

With the industry quickly approaching anarchy, the groundwork was laid for Truman to invoke a Taft-Hartley injunction. Truman swiftly asked Congress for permission to seize control of the mines.[64] Neither the union nor the operators welcomed Truman's move. Miners were unhappy with the prospect of returning to work under the terms of the expired contract after almost a year of working either three days a week or not at all. Operators objected to the prospect of having their operations and profits regulated by the state. Most fundamentally, neither side had faith in the further incursion of government into the industry.[65] Hence, the two sides wasted no time in hammering out their differences. Within hours of Truman's petition, the operators and the union settled their major areas of disagreement. Just two days later, on March 5, 1950, they signed an agreement that was to mark a turning point in the history of labor relations in the coal industry.

The 1950 Compromise and the New Era of Industrial Relations

The National Bituminous Coal Wage Agreement of 1950 marked the coal industry's attempt to craft a strategy to arrest its slide into chaos and restructure itself for enhanced competitiveness. The strategy addressed the signatory operators' two central problems: unreliable production and high costs. Stabilizing production involved quelling the fractious labor relations in the industry. Restoring labor peace was relatively simple: the operators could agree to provide the benefits—chief among them the health and welfare fund—that the miners demanded. While simple, this solution carried a price that was too high given the competition from alternative fuels and small, nonunion operators.

Reestablishing reliable production flows, therefore, had to be coupled with significant reductions in costs in order for union operators to restore their profits in an era of heightened competition. The most effective way to reduce costs was to implement mechanization in the mines to replace the costly, labor-intensive method of mining by hand. Yet the prospect of a wholesale reduction in the mining workforce endangered the union's position. Unfettered mechanization thus threatened to reignite labor strife.

The operators therefore faced a seemingly intractable web of problems. Appeasing labor did not allow operators to meet their lower-cost competitors, while decreasing costs through mechanization increased the risk of inciting labor. However, by 1950, Lewis himself had come to the conclusion that it was in the miners' interest to help rejuvenate the industry. Five years of conflict had not produced a working health or pension plan and the declining prominence of union coal suggested that further conflict was even less likely to yield such benefits.

Lewis also shared the operators' assessment that improving relations between the union and large operators was critical if the industry was to continue to function profitably. By the 1950s, electric utility and steel companies were emerging as the largest consumers of coal and by 1960 would together account for 69 percent of coal consumption (see Table 2). These firms demanded multiyear contracts and reliable, steady supplies of energy.[66] Moreover, utility and steel companies were able to make the investments necessary to switch between fuels in order to achieve these requirements. Obviously, the coal operators could only accommodate these firms with the cooperation of labor and, by 1950, Lewis was willing to cooperate in order to keep jobs in mining.

Lewis's willingness to participate in a strategy that would allow the large union operators to fend off competition from alternative fuels and nonunion mines gave the operators a way out of the web. The settlement reached in 1950 began with the following understanding: the union would agree not to oppose the further introduction of labor-saving mechanization in the mines and, in return, its members would receive enhanced benefits, guaranteed for the long-term. In addition, the agreement inaugurated a new pattern of industrial relations that would require the union to tailor future demands to the health of the industry.[67]

The agreement hinged critically upon the operators' commitment to an employer-financed, union-controlled health and welfare fund. The operators abandoned their attempts to undermine the Fund and agreed to name Josephine Roche as its "neutral" trustee. In effect, this allowed the union, through Lewis and Roche, to control the Fund and ensure its viability. The operators' withdrawal from the management of the Fund would last for more than two decades.

By assuming control of the Fund, the UMWA leadership assured the rank-and-file that the union would direct the efforts to replace the reviled company doctor system. The miners welcomed the union's protection, given that they lacked the knowledge and purchasing power necessary to protect themselves from the potential abuses of a free market in medical care. As a Fund administrator explained,

> To the physician and the hospital administrator, the miner was an outsider. The miner in turn was suspicious, preferring his own crude remedies; a sucker for patent medicines and superstitions. In many things the suspicions were real. The doctor belonged to another world—the country club world, the world of big wheels—a world that defeated his political candidates and furnished hoodlums and strikebreakers to destroy his union.[68]

The miners expected a certain degree of paternalism in the delivery of health benefits and they preferred it to emanate from the union leadership which, in theory at least, was accountable to the beneficiaries of the Fund. Fundamentally, the achievement of quality health benefits was invaluable to miners and their families. As Robert Forrem, a union official in West Virginia noted, "To each and every one of them, the little green photostat card that entitles them to hospitalization is one of their most valued possessions. If you go into their homes, most always you will find this hospitalization card in the covers of the family Bible."[69]

John L. Lewis also realized that the union leadership would benefit from the enhanced rank-and-file loyalty that would result from the UMWA's sponsorship of the health plan. By controlling the plan, Lewis ensured that the Fund was clearly identified with the union. Consequently, the rank-and-file credited the union—and particularly Lewis himself—with the provision of benefits, without acknowledging the operators' role in financing the Fund. The operators understood that allowing the union to take credit for the Fund was a necessary concession to Lewis. The enhanced stature that Lewis obtained as the provider of health benefits put him in a position to accommodate the operators, namely to give his blessing to mechanization. Moreover, there was a flip side to the gains to loyalty that Lewis and the union would realize by providing the benefit; specifically, the Fund would increase the miners' ties to their union, a union that was controlled by a leadership committed to the 1950 agreement.

In return for control of the Fund, Lewis agreed to link the union's demands to the fortunes of the industry in an attempt to strengthen the positions of both the large operators and the union. Most prominently, the union's commitment to increasing productivity was ensured by the linking of the Fund's resources to the industry's output instead of to its payroll. From the time of the Krug-Lewis Accord, the UMWA and the operators agreed to finance the Fund through the assessment of tonnage royalty payments.[70] Interestingly, the type of financing mechanism was almost never a matter of dispute throughout the entire course of negotiations from 1945 to 1950. Lewis suggested a payroll tax only once, during the negotiations in March 1946, that immediately preceded the Krug-Lewis Accord.[71] However, it was the amount, and not the type, of operators' contributions that comprised the bulk of discussions over financing. Initially set at 5 cents per ton in Lewis's 1945 proposal and in the Krug-Lewis Accord, the royalty was increased in each subsequent round of contract talks to 10 cents in 1947, 20 cents in 1949, 30 cents in 1950, and 40 cents in 1952.[72]

The effects of this partnership to implement greater mechanization was evidenced by the decrease in the number of workers and the number of mines in the coal industry (see Table 3). By 1952, employment in the mines in the postwar period dropped to levels that had not been seen since the nineteenth century, heralding a steep decline in mining employment that would continue until the 1970s. Mechanization also hampered the proliferation of small mines. Small mine operators typically were unable to mechanize because of the prohibitively large capital investments required and/or because of the thinness of the veins they excavated. Hence by 1952, the number of mines had begun their decline from their postwar heights back to wartime levels. By 1973, close to 5,000 smaller mines would be eliminated through the combined effects of downturns in demand and competition from large mines with the ability to introduce productivity-enhancing mechanization.[73]

The 1950 contract went beyond crafting a financing mechanism that would align Lewis and the operators on the question of mechanizing the mines. The agreement represented the beginning of a new era of industrial relations in the coalfields. Lewis agreed to a transformation in his role from that of a irascible opponent of management to that of a "labor statesman" dedicated to promoting the vitality of the industry.

Lewis's new perspective manifested itself in several ways. First, after years of turbulence, Lewis did not authorize a single contract strike between 1950 and 1970, nor did he continue to tolerate wildcat strikes. In fact, Lewis imposed fines of $100 a day on locals that chose to strike in defiance of the national union's orders.[74] Second, in the 1950s, Lewis sanctioned a brutal organizing campaign targeting small mines in territory historically inhospitable to organized labor. Under the pretense of an "organizing" drive, the union's aim was to eliminate small mines in order to strengthen the position of the large signatory operators (see chapter 6). Third, Lewis used the union's financial resources to make loans to operators for mechanization and to buy stocks of electric utility companies in order to convince them to buy union coal. Finally, Lewis allowed local unions to enter into sweetheart contracts that permitted operators facing financial difficulty to, among other things, defer their payments to the Fund.

John L. Lewis's decision to promote the attempts of large signatory operators to mechanize the coal industry was a fateful first concession to the forces that would elicit sacrifices from miners throughout the postwar period. Reflecting upon this decision, Lewis often was quoted as saying, "We decided it's better to have half a million men working in the industry at good wages, high standards of living than it is to have a million working in the industry in poverty and degradation."[75] It was a decision that many U.S. labor leaders would face as their industries adapted to the increase in competitive forces after World War II.

Lewis expected many positive consequences to result from the mechanization of the mines. Working miners could look forward to higher pay, better working conditions, quality health benefits, and the security of a pension when they retired. The union would profit from the higher dues that could be assessed on better-paid miners and from the increasing income produced by the tonnage royalty payments to the Fund. A greater percentage of coal would be union-mined as the union would continue to control the jobs in the signatory mines, and the amount of nonunion coal would be reduced through the elimination of small mines unable to mechanize.

It is also possible that Lewis allied the union with the large operators because he was impressed with the relatively better working and living conditions provided by these mines. For example, the industry giant Consolidation Coal Company provided one of the most extensive medical care plans available to miners and their families. Its medical director in Fairmont, West Virginia (about 20 miles southwest of Morgantown), reported to the *American Journal of Public Health* in 1930:

> 163,024 individuals received medical attention . . . typhoid fever and smallpox have been practically eliminated and other communicable diseases materially reduced . . . 50 classes in home hygiene were taught . . . sanitary inspection committees made monthly inspections of most communities . . . the 'Jenkins' Hospital was accepted and accredited by the American College of Surgeons . . . [and] admitted 638 patients for major

illness and injury . . . water and milk supplies were followed up by monthly inspections and laboratory examinations . . . the staff and personnel consisted of 23 full-time, several part-time physicians and 12 public health nurses.[76]

The Boone Report also had reported that large firms and captive mines were more likely to invest in health facilities, reasonable housing stock, and public sanitation for their workforces in order to stabilize production. Large operators were more likely to conclude that caring for workers was, as a report on Inland Steel's mine in Wheelwright, Kentucky, asserted, simply "good business."[77]

For their part, the operators changed their approach to labor relations in order to complement Lewis's contributions. In the months after the 1950 agreement, the northern and captive mine operators formed the Bituminous Coal Operators Association (BCOA). Representing approximately half of the coal mined in the United States, the BCOA dwarfed the unruly Southern Coal Producers Association and its size enabled it to set policy for the entire industry. As it looked toward the 1950s, the BCOA's principal goal was to reduce disruption in the industry (in order to avoid government intervention) and to capture the growing utility market. Specifically, the BCOA sought to replace the industry's intense competition with operator unity designed to prevent a minority group of owners from instigating industry-wide strikes.

The BCOA encouraged its members and Lewis to move away from public, fixed expiration contracts in favor of ongoing, closed-door discussions. Instead of crafting a set of demands each year, or being forced to negotiate with subsets of operators, Lewis would now be able to approach the BCOA when he felt industry conditions would support higher wages and benefits. Consequently, Lewis and his successors negotiated a series of periodic adjustments to the 1950 contract and did not negotiate a completely new contract until 1968.[78]

This new spirit of industrial relations was a startling departure from the status quo in the coal industry, and the BCOA and Lewis wasted no time testing it. In the following two years, Lewis timed his demands to the boost in production spawned by the Korean War, and the BCOA quickly granted two wage increases and an increase in the Fund's royalty rate. Furthermore, in 1953, Lewis successfully negotiated a provision that required signatory operators to pay double the royalty rate on coal they obtained from nonunion mines. Since most of this coal was obtained from small mines that lacked their own cleaning and processing facilities, this provision was intended to reduce the advantages to these mines of remaining nonunion.

The new alliance between Lewis and the BCOA was cemented in 1958 through the formation of the National Coal Policy Conference (NCPC). The

NCPC formally brought together operators, the union, railroads, and major coal consumers. Its first chair was George Love, the head of the Consolidation Coal Corporation, and the driving force behind the formation of the BCOA. In 1962 Love was succeeded, appropriately enough, by John L. Lewis.

The practical effects of the transformation in labor relations in the coal industry were far-reaching. Until the end of the 1940s, the coal industry was governed largely by spot markets. Low barriers to entry and the high demand for coal after the Great Depression resulted in chronic overproduction and intense competition amongst producers. At the same time, the UMWA emerged from the organizing drives made possible by the National Recovery Act as a formidable player in the industry, intent on parlaying its ability to disrupt production during the boom years into advancing the interests of its members.

The often chaotic industrial relations in coal before 1950 proved to be unsustainable with the advent of certain structural changes in the energy markets. Competition from alternative fuels and a decrease in the demand for coal as reconversion drew to a close signaled the end of the rule of King Coal. It had become apparent to both the operators and John L. Lewis that the industry's high costs and instability threatened to drive away irretrievably the electric utilities and steel companies that could return profitability to the coal industry. Moreover, the federal government showed little restraint in directly intervening in coal disputes and dictating settlements that satisfied neither labor nor management.

By agreeing to cut costs through mechanization and enshrine labor stability through the creation of a premium wage and benefit package for workers, the operators and the UMWA leadership replaced the dominance of the spot markets for coal with markets based on long-term contracts. The market for coal became, in effect, two-tiered. Large, mechanized union firms provided fuel for the utilities and industrial firms. Peripheral, nonunion firms supplied coal for the spot markets which remained to furnish coal to smaller consumers and to act as a buffer for demand changes unmet by the long-term contracts. The large mines of the 1940s became even larger in the following decades as BCOA members executed mergers among their own ranks. Market concentration increased markedly as a result. Mines producing over 500 million tons of coal went from providing 35.9 percent of all coal in 1950 to 55.4 percent of all coal in 1975.[79]

The separation of producers into two tiers also served to divide the workforce into two tiers. Mines serving the long-term contract market strived for stable labor relations and, toward that end, paid their workers relatively high wages and provided them with pensions and comprehensive health care. The peripheral mines serving the spot markets could only remain competitive if they kept their labor costs low, given their inability to mechanize, and hence hired workers at low wages without benefits. These mines employed miners unable to obtain jobs in union mines—most often the very miners displaced by the mechanization credited with enhancing the position of their brothers in the BCOA mines.

Lewis never withdrew from the compromise he made in 1950 that installed a new era of labor relations in the coalfields and placed the union squarely on the side of the large operators in a campaign to modernize the industry. He would continue to uphold the agreement even when it became apparent that it involved a number of drawbacks that would haunt the mining workforce in the following decades. First, Lewis had little to offer the thousands of workers who lost their jobs as a result of mechanization and the thousands more who would never have the opportunity to follow their families' footsteps into the mines.[80] Lewis's decision to sacrifice one group of miners for the advancement of another was, in fact, precedent-setting and would be repeated with disturbing frequency in the following decades.

Second, Lewis's approach to the financing of the Fund proved to be successful only when the signatory operators enjoyed healthy production levels. When the industry flourished, the productivity gains provided by mechanization increased the payments to the Fund. However, what Lewis neglected to foresee, or at least underestimated, was the impending drastic decline in the fortunes of the signatory operators. No amount of cooperation from labor could protect the operators from cyclical changes in demand and from their gradual loss of market share to alternative fuels and to nonunion producers utilizing highly productive surface mining methods.

As the traditional bituminous coal mines produced less, the royalty payments to the Fund decreased proportionately. Yet Lewis's conciliatory relationship with the BCOA prevented him from making demands that would have rectified the Fund's precarious financial condition while the industry flagged. For instance, Lewis and the UMWA did not renegotiate the 40 cents per ton royalty rate set in 1952 until 1971. Consequently, the Fund's reserves dipped precipitously, forcing its trustees to match the decrease in income with a decrease in expenditures (see chapter 6).

Finally, Lewis elevated his alliance with the operators to a place of prominence during the remainder of his tenure as president of the UMWA. A particularly striking example occurred at the dedication of the Miners' Memorial Hospitals on June 2, 1956, where Lewis devoted nearly half of his remarks to the gains from the new era of labor-management relations in the industry and the union's responsibility to maintain this labor peace,

> Our industry during the last six years has been living in rather a new era of peace when conflict was abated and when men on both sides of the industry, in immediate positions of leadership, were free to apply themselves to the major project of making this industry successful and making it possible to operate under our system of free enterprise; and today our nation boasts the most efficient, the most productive, coal mining industry in . . . the world. . . . And let me charge each and everyone [sic] of you that only your union can maintain this hospital in its present status and only your union can retain your Welfare Fund. So protect your union and live up to your contract, and discharge your obligations under that contract, so that the operators . . . may have reliance upon your word, and your honor, and the good intent to live up to that obligation when you make your contract. If there are young men among us who are hasty and impulsive, and who have yet failed to achieve and acquire the wisdom that will come to them—I hope—in later years, let the elders of this organization advise them and counsel them and hold them to accountability in your local unions for their wrongful actions.[81]

Because of rain, Lewis cut short his address to the miners and their families who had traveled great distances to attend the dedication of the Miners' Hospitals. Ending on this note, Lewis's dedicatory address resonates more with the admonishment of the potential actions of rebellious rank-and-file than it does with the achievements of the Fund. Placing the Fund at the center of labor relations in coal, just as he did in 1950, Lewis charged the rank-and-file with the task of "cooperating" with management in order to preserve the Fund. Ironically, in the following decades the Fund would be jeopardized not by the actions of the rank-and-file, but rather by the mismanagement and shortsightedness of union leadership under the direction of Lewis himself. It would be the actions of the "rebellious" rank-and-file that would be instrumental in the attempt to save the Fund.

CHAPTER THREE

Designing the Fund

*I*n rallying miners around the demand for employer-financed comprehensive health benefits, John L. Lewis provided few details as to the proposed operation of the new health plan he envisioned. While participants in the events of the late 1940s agreed that the company doctor system was in need of complete overhaul, if not total elimination, few had any sense of the shape of the plan that would replace it. There were simply no precedents for an employer-financed, union-controlled plan of the size and scope Lewis advocated.

The opportunity to create a comprehensive health care plan from the ground up attracted some of the country's most notable health care experts to the design and administration of the project. As one such expert later noted, "It might be said that there are three groups of people in the country who get top super deluxe medical and hospital care; the very poor, the very wealthy and the miners."[1] Bringing miners from the backwater to the forefront of health care provision was an enormous undertaking. Doing so with limited resources made the project much more complicated. Administrators at the Fund quickly discovered that, unlike the very poor and the very wealthy, miners would not be able to utilize unfettered fee-for-service reimbursement for an unlimited range of services if they wanted their plan to survive in the long run.

Fund administrators would become convinced that only through the implementation of managed care initiatives could they attempt to control costs and enhance the quality of services provided to Fund beneficiaries. Yet the administrators would be allowed to direct their efforts only at the provision of specialist and hospital care. The Fund's trustees mandated that the plan be focused on the range of care that enjoyed the highest profile and, as such, provided the greatest and most predictable returns to loyalty from the members.

The tension between political expediency and policy dictates would become a fixture of the Fund's operation. There was perhaps no other decision made by the Fund that displays the consequences of this tension more clearly than the determination to abdicate control over the provision of primary care and center the Fund's efforts on the provision of specialist and hospital care. Emphasizing high-end care would increase its demand and in doing so would undermine the initiatives designed to make the provision of care more cost-effective.

While the Fund's policies evolved over time, its administrative style remained based on continual monitoring and review of provider and beneficiary behavior. As a result, ample documentation exists to describe the motivations behind changes in policy and the results of their implementation. Specifically, the Fund's top administrators left a legacy of letters, memos, unpublished manuscripts, and statistical reports that are now housed in the UMWA Health and Retirement Funds Archives at the West Virginia and Regional History Collection at the West Virginia University Library (Fund Archives), and in the papers of Lorin Edgar Kerr and Robert Kaplan at Yale University (see appendix).

The Launching of the Fund

Rehabilitating the Disabled

As tonnage royalty payments began filling the Fund's coffers in the summer of 1947, the Fund's administrators became anxious to begin reforming the provision of medical care in the coalfields. After a year of turmoil that had included two strikes, the federal government's seizure of the mines, the Centralia disaster, and the publication of the Boone Report, miners had high expectations for improvements in their health care system. Initially, however, the Fund lacked the financial resources necessary to replace the inadequate "check-off" plans with high quality comprehensive care. Thus, instead of delaying the start of benefits until sufficient income was accumulated, the Fund's administrators targeted their efforts at a small but particularly visible and poignant group: the severely disabled.

In 1946 an estimated 50,000 former miners languished bedridden in remote mining communities, disabled by mining accidents and injuries.[2] Rehabilitating these miners fulfilled a dire need and dramatically displayed the Fund's importance. Dr. Howard Rusk, a renowned rehabilitation specialist, saw many of these beneficiaries at the Institute of Physical Medicine and Rehabilitation in New York City:

> These were the toughest cases that anybody ever saw, bar none. You always like to tell about your worst case, but there were many as bad as

this one: this man was 40 years old and his back was broken 20 years before. How he survived that length of time, I don't know. When he was found . . . he . . . had not seen a doctor in 3½ years. There was not even a wagon road to his house and he was carried down in a sling between two bed poles by friends. The man had 11 bed sores from the size of a plate to the size of a dollar; stones in both kidneys and his bladder, and his lower extremities were almost up to his chin. You might ask, is it worth fooling around with a person like that? . . . It took 26 surgical procedures and 13 months before we could even start to train this individual. . . . We trained him to walk . . . on crutches in 90 days, and in control of an automatic bladder and an automatic bowel. And during the last three months of his stay in the Institute, he ran for sheriff in his county . . . and he has been sheriff there for more than three years.[3]

Dr. Rusk's remarks demonstrate the standard elements of the Fund's rehabilitation program. The patient had suffered severe injuries in the mines and had been neglected for a long period of time. Once located by a Fund field representative and approved for rehabilitation, he was transported with the help of his community to a train or plane that would take him to one of the most advanced medical centers in the country, such as the Kessler Rehabilitation Institute in New Jersey, the Institute of Physical Medicine and Rehabilitation in New York, or the Permanente Hospitals in Oakland and Vallejo. Once there, no expense or treatment was spared to rehabilitate the miner, return him to his community, and in many cases, return him to employment. After recovery, the rehabilitated miner became a potent living reminder to his community of the significance of the Fund.

In the first two years of the program, 472 severely handicapped miners received rehabilitation services. More than half of these miners had been injured five or more years earlier. Twenty-four percent entered rehabilitation in a bedfast state and 74 percent entered in wheelchairs; after receiving rehabilitation services, only 6 percent remained bedfast and only 11 percent remained in wheelchairs.[4] The extent of the rehabilitation program's success, while not complete, was striking, particularly given the low expectations Fund beneficiaries had for recovery.

By 1956, a decade after the program's initiation, close to 8,000 severely disabled beneficiaries had been accepted for rehabilitation services.[5] Since more than half were under the age of 45, the Fund also kept track of how many were able to return to the workforce. Of those treated, roughly 3,700, or almost half, were reemployed: 944 returned to the mines, 2,300 found jobs in other industries, and 728 became self-employed.[6] Examining data from the first decade of the program, a Fund report noted that the "typical" beneficiary that returned to employment after rehabilitation was "a 44 year old miner with a back injury. After 16 months of vocational rehabilitation services, he returned to the labor force in a skilled job other than coal-mining, and grossed $63.96 per week or $2,910 annually."[7]

The Fund's rehabilitation program for the severely disabled garnered many awards for its efforts. Specialists at the most prestigious clinics in the country became familiar with the plight of the miners and provided stirring testimonials that drew the attention of the medical community. Dr. Rusk wrote the Fund, "we felt we had been deeply privileged to be a part of this great program of yours that has given help to the helpless and hope to the hopeless."[8] The Fund spent roughly five years and over $4.5 million on the intensive rehabilitation of disabled Fund beneficiaries.[9] By the mid-1950s, the rehabilitation program had achieved its dual objectives: to rehabilitate the large backlog of disabled miners, and to establish the Fund's reputation in the minds of its beneficiaries as a plan that provided service of unparalleled quality for even the most neglected workers.

The Administration and Structure of the Fund

Soon after the 1948 contract was signed, Josephine Roche, the trustee designated director of the Fund, began recruiting staff for the Fund. Heeding the advice of the health care professionals she consulted, Roche recruited administrators and physicians who shared a willingness to participate in the innovative policies necessary to create the health plan envisioned by the union. The size of the undertaking alone, providing care for almost two million beneficiaries, made it a daunting project. The added ambition of providing quality, comprehensive care in areas lacking adequate medical personnel and facilities—so vividly documented in the Boone Report of the preceding year—made the task positively formidable. Such a venture required the commitment of a staff dedicated to reforming completely the substandard system of medical care.

Roche's first step was to recruit a staff to coordinate the overall administration of the Fund from its national office in Washington, D.C. Based on her experience supervising the U.S. Public Health Service in the 1930s, Roche was convinced that it was "vital . . . to have well-trained experts to administer the medical program."[10] To direct the Washington office, Roche hired Dr. Warren F. Draper as the Fund's medical director. Draper proved to be an uncannily good choice to head the Fund's medical operations. Having served capably in various executive positions in the American Medical Association, Draper came to the Fund with a solid conservative reputation. Draper's stature gave the Fund a measure of legitimacy in health care circles that proved to be invaluable when the Fund eventually deviated significantly from established patterns of care.

Interestingly, despite his conservative reputation, Draper proved to be surprisingly accommodating in allowing his staff to develop the innovative practices that would distinguish the Fund. As Albert Deutsch commented: "Dr. Draper's loyalty to organized medicine was surpassed only by his passionate devotion to the principle of 'high quality medicine for Americans at fair and reasonable cost.'"[11] Throughout his twenty-year tenure as the Fund's medical director, Draper effectively managed to capitalize on his conservative credentials while encouraging his staff to engage in innovations outside the mainstream of medical care provision.[12]

One of the hallmarks of the Fund's administration was its monitoring of the quality and cost-effectiveness of care at the local level. Given the dispersion of beneficiaries across the United States, the Fund's staff felt that only an inadequate amount of administrative supervision could be exercised from the national office in Washington. Thus, most of the responsibility for daily operations was delegated to ten Area Medical Offices (AMOs) positioned throughout the coalfields to better respond to local needs. As Dr. Draper summarized:

> Conditions differ widely over the far-flung area in which the mining communities are situated. The density of population, geographic location, proximity to medical centers, number and character of hospitals, the number of physicians in relation to the number of people and their distribution, the types of services that can be provided adequately—all present individual problems that require careful study to find the solution best suited to the area in which they exist.[13]

While the bulk of administrative operations were transferred to the AMOs, the national office retained ultimate authority in decision-making. For example, invoices for medical services received by the AMOs were transferred to Washington for audit and payment (see below). Data collected by the AMOs were forwarded to the national office for review. Finally, decisions made by the AMOs, such as those concerning eligibility and treatment authorization, could be appealed to the Fund's national office.

The Fund established AMOs based on the location of beneficiaries in the late 1940s (see Map 1). Eight of the ten AMOs served beneficiaries in the Appalachian coal basin: three offices opened in West Virginia at Beckley, Morgantown, and Charleston; two offices opened in Pennsylvania at Pittsburgh (also serving Ohio) and Johnstown; two offices opened at Knoxville and Louisville to serve Tennessee, eastern Kentucky, and western Virginia; and an office opened in Birmingham to serve Alabama beneficiaries. The two remaining AMOs served the coalfields west of Appalachia. The St. Louis AMO served beneficiaries in the Interior Basin coalfields of Illinois, Iowa, Missouri, Kansas, Oklahoma, and Arkansas.[14] Finally, the Denver AMO served beneficiaries in the Western Basin coalfields primarily located in Colorado, Montana, Wyoming, New Mexico, Utah, Washington, and Alaska.

By December 1948, each Area Medical Office had recruited its own administrative and technical staff, as well as a physician administrator to head its operations (see Figure 1). The AMOs performed three basic functions: they administered payments, reviewed the cost and quality of care supplied by providers in their area, and procured public monies for the treatment of eligible beneficiaries. The Fund's payment system almost exclusively was limited to a series of exchanges between the Fund and providers. Beneficiaries were issued identification cards ("health cards") which they presented to their physicians upon receiving treatment. Physicians would then send an invoice for the treatment provided to the AMO. The AMO staff would review the invoice and make note of the cost and the treatment provided. Within 48 hours, the AMO would forward the bill to the Washington office for audit and payment. If a physician recommended hospitalization, the beneficiary would be given a note to be filed with the local union stating the reasons hospitalization was deemed necessary. The local would then issue a hospitalization slip which would be returned to the physician ensuring that payment would be received for services rendered in the hospital.[15] Payment for these services was obtained in the same manner as for physician care.

Another important task of the Fund offices was the procurement of public monies for eligible beneficiaries in order to reduce Fund outlays. For example, the Fund directed beneficiaries to county health departments for treatment of tuberculosis and venereal disease, and for cancer control programs. The Fund transferred beneficiaries diagnosed with polio to Crippled Children's Services and the National Foundation for Infant Paralysis for treatment.[16] The Fund supplemented its treatment of disabled beneficiaries with services obtained from public vocational rehabilitation programs. Finally, the Fund helped disabled miners apply for Federal Old Age and Survivors Disability Insurance (OASDI); by 1972, approximately 25,000 former miners had enrolled in this program.[17]

Map 1 Location of Area Medical Offices and their areas of jurisdiction

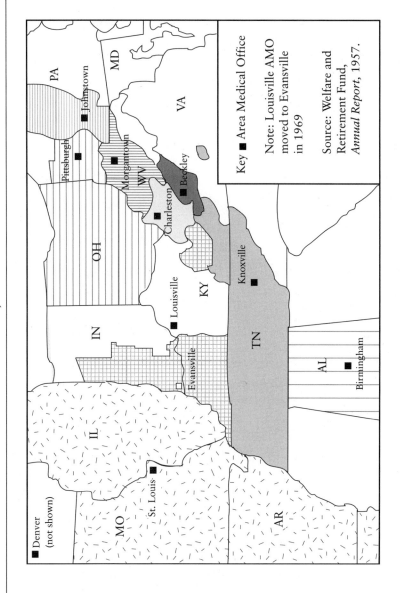

Key ■ Area Medical Office

Note: Louisville AMO moved to Evansville in 1969

Source: Welfare and Retirement Fund, *Annual Report*, 1957.

Figure 1 Organizational chart (selected portions), UMWA Welfare and
Retirement Funds, 1961

Trustees
John L. Lewis, Chairman and Chief Executive Officer
Josephine Roche
Henry Schmidt

Director
Josephine Roche

Executive Medical Officer
Warren Draper

Deputy Executive Medical Officer
John Morrison

Area Medical Offices

Beckley	*Knoxville*
Deane Brooke	John Winebrenner
Birmingham	*Louisville*
Allen Koplin	Asa Barnes
Charleston	*Morgantown*
William Riheldaffer	Hubert Marshall
Denver	*Pittsburgh*
William Dorsey	Leslie Falk
Johnstown	*St. Louis*
F. H. Arestad	George Brother

Miners Memorial Hospital Association
John Newdorp, Medical Administrator

Research Director
Robert Kaplan

Source: UMWA, Welfare and Retirement Fund, *Annual Report* (Washington, D.C.: UMWA,
1961), 8–9.

It is interesting to note that while in principle the UMWA eschewed provision of care by the state, in practice it aggressively sought state services for certain beneficiaries. This contradiction is explained by noting the composition of the beneficiary groups involved and the type of care they received. First, the treatment required by the very ill and disabled was often tremendously costly. By allowing state and federal agencies to pay for this treatment, the Fund avoided making payments that would have significantly curtailed the amount of funds available to provide other services. Second, the groups that were transferred to state agencies were a small proportion of the total beneficiary pool and a marginal constituency within the union. The Fund continued to be the sole health care plan for the vast majority of working and retired miners and their families who, as a result, remained indebted by extension to the union. Moreover, the fact that the Fund typically was instrumental in helping beneficiaries apply for these services meant that it was still in some way associated with the state aid beneficiaries received. In effect, then, by transferring a small group of marginal beneficiaries to state care, the UMWA did not lose an appreciable amount of the returns to loyalty that accrue from the provision of care.

Finally, the Fund prided itself on the administrative efficiency it achieved as a self-insured plan. Administrative costs remained below 3 percent of expenditures each year in its first two decades of operation. A significant portion of the savings were reaped from the financing of the plan. Fund royalties were received directly from operators and the Fund, unlike mainstream insurers, did not have the overhead associated with sales, marketing, and premium collection. In addition, the Fund claimed to be more efficient than typical insurers because of its ability to tailor its services to the needs of its beneficiaries through the coordination of the area and national offices.[18]

It is important to note that attention to organizational efficiency was only part of the Fund's overall approach to provider review. Equally important was the spirit of this review. As a physician noted in a letter to the Fund's executive medical officer in 1959,

> I doubt very much whether you realize the value of your contribution, and of the change you are making in medicine and the social order. I have been laboring in this section of the Lord's vineyard for more than forty years. By far the most pleasant association I have had in this long period has been with the men who work under your direction. I have never know these men to be anything but honorable, just and true, vitally interested in the common good. I do not like over-worked words such as dedicated, concerned, or consecrated, but these men associated with you are dedicated souls in the real sense of the term. If I had to go back to

the old order of things, I doubt whether I would have the courage to carry on.[19]

The sentiments expressed in this letter are a far cry from the criticisms physicians typically level at administrators who review their operations. The Fund attempted to facilitate the departures it made from the mainstream by placing close attention not only to the design of its innovations, but also to their implementation.

The Initial Period of Operation: 1948–1949

The Fund had enjoyed only eight months of operations before its trustees were forced to suspend benefits in September of 1949. The Fund's coffers were depleted quickly once southern operators refused to make royalty payments after the 1949 contract expired in July (see chapter 2). While miners struck throughout the fall of 1949 and into the next year to protest the operators' actions, the Fund's administrators turned their attention toward reviewing the experience of the first months of the plan's operation. This period of review and reflection revealed that while more beneficiaries received more care from more providers, the care they received was not necessarily of adequate quality and certainly was not cost-effective. This outcome is not surprising given the incentives for overutilization inherent in a plan combining fee-for-service reimbursement with comprehensive coverage. This ten-month hiatus until the Fund resumed operation proved to be critical in changing the approach of its staff. During this respite, administrators evaluated the Fund's initial period of operation and became convinced that the problems of overutilization and low quality care could only be remedied through reforms that transformed the Fund into a plan guided by managed care principles.

The need to initiate programs quickly after the 1948 contract was signed did not allow the Fund's administrators to give much attention to controlling the costs or the quality of care received by beneficiaries. As Warren Draper explained:

Here we were with money coming in and members of course knowing about Mr. Lewis' desire to have this Fund for his people, and naturally they want care without having to wait any great length of time. They wanted medical care right now and not six months from now. The problem was to provide it right now and the only way to do it was to use the facilities in existence. You have hospitals of certain kinds around these coal mining areas, and some doctors, and you develop a plan to use these people to the best advantage you can.[20]

During its first eight months of operation, the Fund reimbursed providers on a fee-for-service basis for all medical treatments. Subsequent reviews by the AMOs of the cost and provision of care based on the invoices received from providers revealed widespread abuses of the plan. Administrators identified three major sources of abuse: the fee-for-service reimbursement method, the heavy use of substandard medical infrastructure, and the unrestricted scope of care provided to beneficiaries.

The most common problem uncovered by the AMOs was the performance of unnecessary treatments which the Fund then reimbursed on a fee-for-service basis. It appeared that a significant number of providers viewed the Fund as "an inexhaustible grab-bag."[21] For example, a pathologist's report at one hospital showed appendicitis in only 25 out of 45 appendectomies performed.[22] The Fund's liberal reimbursement policies appear to have exacerbated the situation. Administrators discovered that the rate of appendectomies in areas with large mining populations had been more than twice the rates in contiguous non-mining areas.[23] The AMOs discovered that many physicians had used antibiotics excessively and that some physicians had exaggerated the severity of their patients' illnesses in order to be able to "treat" them longer.[24] The AMOs also found that excessive hospitalization was common at closed-staff proprietary hospitals that urged their doctors to fill empty beds. Moreover, the quality of care in many of these hospitals was dubious as they lacked the equipment and personnel necessary to achieve listings with the American Hospital Association or the American Medical Association.[25]

Upon review of their records, the AMOs also found that physicians often billed the Fund for treatment that was not even performed. For instance, the Fund was sometimes charged for the care of patients who had already been discharged.[26] By reviewing the accumulated invoices, the AMOs also compared the charges of physicians over time and in relation to each other, and revealed instances of excessive charges. While the vast majority of physicians apparently provided "honest, conscientious and competent service," the minority that abused the Fund's reimbursement policy created "substantial, significant, and decisive" problems.[27]

Finally, the Fund's administrators noticed that its unrestricted reimbursement plan spawned moral hazard on the part of beneficiaries. In eliminating the lack of freedom of choice of physician—the most egregious aspect of the company doctor system—the Fund swung to the other extreme and allowed beneficiaries to seek care from any physician.[28] As a result, the AMOs discovered that, given the opportunity to receive care from any of the many physicians eager to treat them, the Fund's beneficiaries tended to over-utilize medical services of questionable quality.[29] Concurrently, the number of physicians willing to treat miners and their families increased as physicians were lured to the coalfields by the prospect of securing the lucrative practices made possible by the Fund. What made this influx even more troubling was that many of these physicians were of dubious caliber. For instance, in a section of eastern Kentucky, 11 out of 36 practitioners were over 70 years of age, two were known drug addicts, three were practicing under limited licenses, and two had not graduated from medical school.[30] Given the extent of physician shortages throughout the coalfields, the Fund had no choice but to use these physicians.

Concerned that unchecked, the abuses of the Fund could threaten the plan's long-term viability, the Fund's administrators turned their attention to crafting reforms to address the problems of substandard infrastructure, excessive utilization, and unreasonable charges. Two factors made these reforms possible: the Fund's significance as a payer in local markets and administrators' commitment to managed care principles.

First, the Fund's size and self-insured character fulfilled an important prerequisite for implementing extensive reform. The Fund's significance as a payer in local markets allowed it to dictate administrative policies and reimbursement guidelines. Providers that relied extensively on the business generated by Fund beneficiaries had little choice but to adhere to the Fund's directives. Moreover, the Fund could promote reforms directly instead of working through a third-party insurer.

Table 5 demonstrates the relative size of the Fund's beneficiary pool in relation to each local area's total beneficiary pool beginning in 1955, the earliest date for which this information is available.[31] Not surprisingly, Fund beneficiaries comprised a significantly higher percentage of hospital patients in Appalachia than anywhere else in the United States. The first reason for this pattern is that the comparative size of the mining population was greater in Appalachia than in urban areas like Pittsburgh and Johnstown or than in areas producing relatively less coal like those represented by the St. Louis and Denver AMOs. Second, the Fund's prominence in Appalachia was also due to the general population's lack of access, both physical and financial, to medical care in this region. It should be noted that the declining importance of the Fund over time suggested in Table 5 was a result of changes in both

Table 5 Hospital admissions and days of care of Fund beneficiaries as a percentage of each AMO's total admissions and days of care, 1955–1970

Area	Admissions					Days of Care				
	1955[a]	1960[a]	1965	1970	average[b] 1955–1970	1955[a]	1960[a]	1965	1970	average[b] 1955–1970
Beckley	36.1%	17.3%	18.3%	15.5%	19.6%	39.2%	16.3%	19.3%	12.7%	18.7%
Charleston	17.4	19.6	11.9	10.9	15.0	20.8	22.7	15.5	10.9	16.5
Morgantown	13.2	11.7	8.0	9.5	10.8	15.7	15.4	9.7	10.2	13.2
Knoxville	9.3	5.6	2.7	3.6	5.3	11.0	7.2	4.0	3.2	5.7
Birmingham	6.1	5.1	2.2	2.8	3.6	10.9	6.2	2.6	3.0	4.7
Louisville	8.6	5.0	1.1	1.8	3.8	9.1	5.0	1.3	1.7	3.8
Johnstown	5.8	5.8	2.4	1.8	4.4	7.8	8.3	3.1	4.6	6.0
Pittsburgh	1.8	1.5	1.1	1.5	1.5	2.5	2.2	1.5	1.7	2.0
St. Louis	2.0	1.5	0.9	1.5	1.4	2.2	1.7	1.2	1.2	1.5
Denver	1.1	0.9	0.6	0.7	0.8	1.4	1.2	0.7	0.8	1.0
ALL AREAS	5.3%	4.2%	2.3%	3.2%	3.6%	5.9%	4.9%	2.7%	3.1%	4.0%

[a] Includes data from Miners Memorial Hospitals (see chapter 6.)
[b] Averages are computed using annual data for all years between 1955 and 1970.

Source: UMWA Welfare and Retirement Fund, Office of Research and Statistics, "Hospital Service to Fund Beneficiaries," various years, Fund Archives.

these factors; the size of the Fund's beneficiary pool decreased as the mining population decreased, and the general population's use of medical care increased as their access to care increased.

Table 6 provides an even closer look at the importance of the Fund by displaying the proportion of hospital services used by Fund beneficiaries in selected hospitals in the Beckley AMO. It should be noted that the high concentration of miners in the Beckley area made the Fund a more significant in payer here than in any other area, with the result that the data presented in Table 6 are not necessarily characteristic of the standard experience of hospitals that served Fund beneficiaries. In 1955, the earliest year that these data are available, eight hospitals—among the largest in the Beckley area—attributed at least roughly a third of their admissions and days of care to Fund beneficiaries. Among this group, three hospitals—Wyoming General, Grace and Beckley Hospitals—all had a patient base that was comprised of roughly 60 percent Fund beneficiaries. Moreover, these hospitals were spread throughout the Beckley area so that the impact of the Fund was felt over a wide geographic range. The prominence of the Fund decreased over time in Beckley as in all areas, but by 1970, there were still five hospitals that derived more than 20 percent of their admissions and patient days from Fund beneficiaries.[32]

Second, bolstered by their relative power in local medical markets, Fund administrators realized that they were in a position to promote reforms consonant with their progressive beliefs. Their interest in managed care compelled administrators to eschew minor adjustments to the operation of the Fund. Instead, the Fund promulgated a series of major reforms that fundamentally altered traditional patterns of care and reimbursement for Fund beneficiaries. In brief, the Fund's efforts were designed to achieve two ends: a reduction in the overutilization of medical services and an improvement in the quality of personnel and facilities available to beneficiaries. It is important to note the tension between these two objectives—namely, that increased quality of care will lead to an increase in the demand for care in the absence of utilization controls.

In short, the Fund's first eight months of operation provided the administrators with useful experience in operating a health plan of unprecedented size and scale. During this initial period, over 26,000 beneficiaries received care from 6,500 physicians and 600 hospitals at a cost of over $4.7 million.[33] Albert Deutsch summarized:

> This industry-wide program, covering more than one million persons with a complete medical, hospital and dental care plan, was by far the most

Table 6 Short-term hospital admissions to and days of care of Fund beneficiaries as a percentage of each hospital's total admissions and days of care, selected hospitals in the Beckley AMO, 1955–1970

Location	Hospital	Admissions				Days of Care			
		1955	1960	1965	1970	1955	1960	1965	1970
Oak Hill, WV	Oak Hill Hospital	59.1%	37.5%	21.1%		56.4%	42.5%	25.4%	
Mullens, WV	Wyoming General Hospital	58.8	49.2	36.2	43.0	62.1	56.3	39.4	40.9
Welch, WV	Grace Hospital	57.3	42.5	50.5		61.5	64.0	52.1	
Beckley, WV	Beckley Hospital	47.2	20.4	10.4	33.0	57.1	27.1	10.7	10.1
Welch, WV	Stevens Clinic Hospital	46.6	45.7	36.6	42.1	53.1	45.8	37.1	38.2
Beckley, WV	Raleigh General Hospital	42.0	21.0	9.5	20.3	50.0	25.6	8.9	20.2
Bluefield, WV	Bluefield Sanitarium	33.4	21.4	17.4	18.8	37.7	27.0	26.8	17.8
Bluefield, WV	St. Lukes Hospital	30.5	24.5	16.6	21.8	32.3	29.0	18.4	19.1
Princeton, WV	Mercer Memorial Hospital	17.7	14.4	8.9		23.5	16.5	13.5	
Ronceverte, WV	Greenbrier Valley Hospital	14.6	9.0	7.1	6.1	17.4	9.9	7.5	5.3
Hinton, WV	Hinton Hospital	9.9	4.7	2.1	3.4	10.5	5.4	1.8	2.5
Beckley, WV	Beckley Memorial Hospital[a]		78.4	62.3	45.0		83.1	67.4	43.7
	Beckley AMO Totals	36.1%	17.3%	18.3%	15.5%	39.2%	16.3%	19.3%	12.7%

[a] Beckley Memorial Hospital was operated directly by the Fund until 1964 when it was sold to Appalachian Regional Hospitals, Inc. (see chapter 6).

Source: Office of Research and Statistics, "Hospital Service to Fund Beneficiaries," various years, Fund Archives.

comprehensive experiment of its kind ever to be attempted for a civilian population in the U.S. It began auspiciously, with the bravos and huzzahs of organized medicine tingling in the ears of its creators. It proved short-lived; the experiment was aborted in its ninth month, almost wrecking the UMWA Fund. It left Dr. Draper and his associates sadder and wiser men. Within those nine months, they gained a wealth of experience and knowledge that enabled them later to build sturdily on the ruins of a noble experiment in undisciplined and inadequately controlled medicine.[34]

The respite provided by the suspension of benefits as the 1950 agreement was hammered out allowed the Fund's administrators to examine the quality and cost of care provided in the coalfields. The unsatisfactory results they found reinforced the need for extensive reforms and provided the impetus for the transformation of the Fund into a system based on managed care.

The Priority of Political Objectives and the Reshaping of the Fund

When health benefits resumed on July 1, 1950, after the signing of the historic 1950 contract, both beneficiaries and providers found that they would no longer enjoy completely unrestricted access to the Fund. Fund administrators had begun the process of implementing reforms that were designed to eliminate the abuses spawned by unfettered fee-for-service reimbursement for a virtually unlimited range of services provided by, in many instances, substandard providers.

The administrators had two basic objectives in the reform of the Fund. First, administrators sought to improve the access to and quality of care available to beneficiaries. Second, in part to have the funds available to achieve the first objective, the administrators sought to make the provision of care more cost-effective. As extensive and innovative as the administrators' reforms would be, they were aimed almost exclusively at the delivery and financing of specialist and hospital care. When the Fund resumed operation in 1950, primary care was no longer covered. While many Fund beneficiaries continued to have access to primary care through check-off plans, the inability of Fund administrators to directly control this range of care ultimately would affect their ability to achieve their objectives.

At first glance it may seem curious that administrators who championed comprehensive managed care would allow the provision of primary care to fall outside their purview. In fact, over the course of the following decades, many administrators lamented the exclusion of primary care from the plan's coverage. However, the decision on whether or not to include primary care was not guided solely by the health policy aims of the administrators. Rather, the impetus for focusing the Fund's finances and energies on specialist and hospital care emanated from the political imperatives mandated by the union's leadership.

John L. Lewis's primary goal in bargaining for the Fund was to mobilize miner loyalty and thereby strengthen the UMWA. Lewis and Josephine Roche, the union's trustees on the Fund's board, believed that this goal would be best achieved by ensuring that the Fund maintained a high profile. They were instrumental in promoting the high visibility projects the Fund became known for: the rehabilitation of the severely disabled, the abolition of the widely reviled company doctor system, and the provision of services like hospital and specialist care most noticeably lacking in the coalfields.

The trustees' vision did not leave much room for the administrators' desire to finance routine care and engage in lower profile managed care exercises. The trustees did not consider these initiatives to be as potent in terms of increasing the association of the Fund with the union in the minds of miners and their families. In addition, the trustees had misgivings about providing primary care after the Fund's brief experiment with comprehensive coverage in 1948 and 1949 had nearly ruined the Fund financially. Yet even after the Fund instituted better controls, reduced its use of fee-for-service reimbursement, and benefited from the development of the medical care infrastructure in the coalfields, the trustees still did not sanction coverage of routine care on more than a limited basis.

The trustees failed to foresee, however, the inherent tension between their vision of the Fund's mission and the changes in industry structure Lewis helped fashion beginning in 1950. First, the high profile, high quality, hospital-based system promoted by the trustees increased the demand for specialist and hospital services with the result that total costs as well as the cost per beneficiary increased. Second, the process of mechanization that was allowed to accelerate—as a concession for the Fund—produced a beneficiary pool that placed significant demands on the health care system beyond the already formidable ones posed by this particular population.

At the same time as these two forces served to raise costs, the financing mechanism designed in 1950 proved to be incapable of generating either the levels or the stability of income necessary to fund the program envisioned by the trustees. Most notably, as the industry experienced a fall in demand in the late 1950s and early 1960s, the Fund experienced a reduction in income just as it began its most expensive and high profile undertaking—the operation of its own chain of hospitals. Moreover, the pay-as-you-go nature of the financing mechanism produced operating deficits that had to be offset by immediate reductions in expenditures. The cost-control initiatives implemented by the administrators generally were not able to rectify these deficits as most were designed to produce savings only in the long term. As a result, the trustees were forced to limit the Fund's programs either in duration or in scope, or to limit the size of the beneficiary pool. The inadequacies of the financing mechanism forced the trustees to take actions that undermined not only the initiatives of administrators, but also, ironically, their own attempts to elevate the Fund's stature in the eyes of beneficiaries.

The first major reform of Fund policy was a reduction in the scope of services it covered. The most significant change was the elimination of coverage for general practitioner home and office care.[35] It is important to note that this did not mean that beneficiaries were in all cases denied access to care, but that the Fund gave up control over this dimension of care. There are frequent references to the fact that miners continued the practice of check-off arrangements for the immunizations, minor medications, and routine home and office visits that the Fund no longer covered. While evidence of the prevalence and operation of these plans is incomplete, it appears that the vast majority of miners participated in these now voluntary plans where they existed. Employers generally administered the plans for working miners, and local unions handled the plans for retired miners and widows.[36] For example, the Russellton Clinic received a check-off of $4.00 per month for working miners with families, $3.00 for unmarried working miners and married retired miners, $2.00 for single retired miners, and $0.50 for widows.[37] The adverse consequences of the Fund's elimination of coverage for routine care was mitigated, then, by the fact that many miners continued to be insured for this care.

However, even where check-off plans did exist, the incentives embodied in the Fund's reimbursement for specialist and hospital care often continued to generate inappropriate care. Morgantown area administrator Herbert Marshall noted,

> the check-off physician . . . rather than going to the trouble of providing adequate care in the home or office, relieves himself of some problem patients by referring them unnecessarily to specialist for care at the Fund's expense. The same thing is true for fee-for-service general practitioner when he feels that he will probably not be paid for his services, he refers the patient to a specialist for treatment at Fund expense rather than spend his time in caring for the patient.[38]

Fund administrators were keenly aware of the incentive providers faced to charge the Fund for specialist or hospital care instead of forgoing Fund reimbursement and providing less expensive primary care. As Marshall summarized, "Our present program is a hospital program; we pay for services in the hospital so the incentive for both physician and patient is for hospitalization."[39]

Area administrators, in fact, frequently lobbied for a reinstatement of coverage of routine primary care, especially once the AMOs were in a better position to monitor the care provided. In 1955 Marshall noted, "Frankly, we are convinced that a complete medical program with the general practitioner as a full time partner on the medical team would not be as expensive as our partial program."[40] Fund administrators finally got a chance to test this claim in the early 1960s when the Fund approved a set of pilot Medical Management programs that extended primary care coverage to a limited number of beneficiaries. The AMOs sponsored two basic types of Medical Management programs. In regions with established group practices and concentrated beneficiary pools, beneficiaries enrolled in Medical Management programs at the clinics for complete comprehensive care. In regions where group practices were not as prevalent and/or where beneficiaries were geographically dispersed, AMOs used funds available under the Medical Management program to improve outpatient services and/or to enroll only narrowly-defined groups like the chronically ill and the elderly in comprehensive care programs.

While the design of the Medical Management programs is fairly well documented,[41] little is known about the impact of the programs after the initial period of operation. It is likely that the Medical Management experiment turned out to fulfill the expectations of Deane Brooke, the area medical administrator for the Beckley AMO:

> To initiate such a program *now* based on the assumption that it will immediately diminish costs to the Fund seems overly optimistic and perhaps unrealistic. Hasn't the experience been that new and better services usually increase utilization for a while? There is no question in my mind that it will decrease costs in the future but how soon and in what manner can only be determined through experimentation.[42]

Brooke had identified the inherent tension between the Fund's desire to increase the quality of its coverage while reducing costs: the higher demand that was likely to result from the increase in quality would only decrease costs if the Fund's other policies reduced the potential for unnecessary care.

In addition to the termination of coverage for home and office care, the Fund promulgated further restrictions in coverage designed to target other abuses of the Fund. First, to reduce excessive prescription of drugs, the Fund eliminated coverage for drugs for acute care and continued to cover only expensive drugs needed on a long-term basis (e.g., insulin). Again, check-off plans for routine care typically included coverage for minor prescription drugs. Second, the Fund eliminated coverage for tonsillectomies and adenoidectomies once it discovered that these procedures were routinely prescribed by physicians who failed to determine whether, in fact, they were absolutely necessary.

Third, hospitalization and other services prescribed solely for the treatment of acute alcoholism also were eliminated from the plan's coverage. This restriction appears to have emanated more from concerns over the "morality" of covering care for alcoholics than from a desire to reduce costs.[43] Fourth, the Fund eliminated routine dental services from the plan, and continued to cover only those dental procedures that were prescribed as part of an hospitalized illness. Finally, the Fund eliminated coverage for compensable injuries that were the responsibility of an employer through the Workmen's Compensation Fund.[44] This policy complemented the administrators' drive to find alternative sources of funds to care for certain eligible groups.

The restrictions on coverage when the Fund resumed operations in 1950 served to focus the Fund on the specialist and hospital care that its trustees were most interested in providing. While the Fund lamentably would lose direct control over the provision of primary care, the administrators were reassured by the fact that the vast majority of miners still had access to this care through affordable check-off plans. It is interesting to note that the Fund did not promote more typical cost-saving incentives like co-payments and deductibles. The Fund considered it inappropriate to attempt to influence patients' behavior given their lack of the medical knowledge needed to assess whether a prescribed course of treatment was appropriate.[45] The Fund's position on this issue again placed it outside the mainstream of developments in the financing of medical care.

The Consequences of Emphasizing Specialist and Hospital Care

Overall, the Fund's efforts to provide health care to miners and their families would be concentrated almost exclusively on the provision of specialist and hospital care. With the exception of the limited Medical Management programs, routine care was not covered by the Fund after 1950. As a result, beneficiaries received this care under check-off plans out of the direct control of the Fund or went without primary care altogether. The Fund did improve the access to and quality of primary care physicians by recruiting them to practices in the coalfields and by reimbursing the doctors for the specialist and hospital care (as attending physicians) that they provided. However, beyond this indirect contribution to the provision of primary care, the Fund did little to encourage beneficiaries to seek routine care or to encourage physicians to provide this care when necessary.

The failure of the Fund to promote appropriate levels of primary care would adversely affect its ability to increase the cost-effectiveness of care. Beneficiaries who lacked coverage for routine care had no incentive to seek care until specialist or hospital care could be obtained and covered by the Fund. Physicians had few pecuniary incentives to treat beneficiaries early since the Fund reimbursed them only for providing specialist and hospital care. The Fund did have some safeguards, albeit imperfect, against excessive exploitation of this arrangement. The AMOs' review of physician care prevented physicians from charging the Fund for care that should have been provided on a routine basis. In addition, the Medical Management programs sponsored by the AMOs in the early 1960s created incentives for physicians to provide more primary care.

The Fund had eliminated the coverage of routine care from its program as part of its general overhaul in 1950 to reduce the tremendous costs associated with unfettered use of primary care physicians. Yet the savings realized from this decision did not result in a proportionate reduction in *total* costs. Savings in primary care would be offset by increases in the cost of specialist and hospital care that resulted from the incentives faced by beneficiaries and physicians to seek such care. This outcome impeded the Fund's ability to increase the cost-effectiveness of care.

The incentives beneficiaries and providers faced to engage in early, primary care were even weaker when viewed in relation to the prominence of the specialist and hospital component of the Fund program. As will be discussed in chapters 4 and 5, the Fund sponsored an unprecedented increase in the access to specialist and hospital care by recruiting physicians to the coalfields, developing group practices, and building hospitals. The Fund also enhanced the quality of care by limiting reimbursement to qualified physicians, reviewing physician practices, educating providers, and underwriting the modernization and expansion of hospitals. The Fund's efforts did not go unnoticed by beneficiaries who paid no fee for specialist and hospital care.

As early as 1952, Warren Draper noted that these high profile endeavors to improve access to and quality of care lead to higher use:

> It is a fact that the need for more medical care by the Fund instead of less is being indicated. More people are becoming eligible, more eligibles are taking advantage of their opportunity, more confidence in the benefits to be derived has been engendered. These are the most important factors in adding to the increasing demand and cost.[46]

Hubert Marshall, the chief administrator for the Morgantown AMO, expanded:

> The satisfactory effective treatment to patients in the hospital is soon known throughout the immediate vicinity. . . . more and more people become interested in good medical care and identify it as necessary for healthful living. . . . These people never attempted to understand the operation of a hospital and how they could help increase the medical services in order to benefit themselves. We feel that the Fund has helped change these thoughts so that more of the community works to maintain modern, efficient hospital care.[47]

The desire of beneficiaries to receive high quality care was complemented by the incentives the Fund afforded physicians to provide this care. Physicians were reimbursed for specialist and hospital services and were encouraged to provide as much of it as necessary. Marshall commented,

> [Miners] are no longer poor relatives whose medical needs are postponed, delayed, shunted aside and frequently ignored. . . . A punster referred to him recently as the unwanted child suddenly declared legitimate. He is sought after and pursued. After years on a starvation medical diet, he is the principal guest at the feast and his dietary problem is no longer that of insufficiency, but super-abundance . . .
>
> Doctors have available every facility of modern medicine with which to treat our patients. They have practically operated carte blanche with unlimited freedom. Every incentive has been offered to do more and better work. As a result, the miner has received more medical care than a member of any group of which we have knowledge. There have been more hospital admissions, more hospital days, greater use of . . . E.K.G.'s, etc., more surgery, greater use of drugs, etc. than for any group of people in our country; *but therein was also our greatest problem*.[48]

Marshall had identified the fundamental problem inherent in the Fund's bias toward the provision of high-end care: not only did total costs increase, but the cost per beneficiary also rose in the absence of coverage for routine care. This problem was exacerbated by characteristics of the mining regions and the mining population. First, the lack of appropriate facilities and qualified physicians in the mining regions hampered the ability of the AMOs to administer the provision of care in the most cost-effective manner. As early as 1952, Warren Draper noted that decreases in expenditures were only likely to occur as better facilities and personnel became available that would allow care to be provided outside of hospitals.[49] Hospitalization rates were high where diagnostic and ambulatory services could only be provided on an inpatient basis. This problem would recede over time as hospital services expanded to include outpatient services and physicians established clinics that provided diagnostic services.[50]

Administrators also found that high hospitalization rates arose not only where there were insufficient substitutes, but also where there was excess hospital capacity. For instance, Denver administrators cited the oversupply of hospital beds in its AMO as the major culprit in the overutilization of hospital services:

> As nature abhors a vacuum, hospital administrators and physicians abhor empty hospital beds. . . . The availability of hospital beds in some communities has changed the whole pattern of medical practice, to the extent that any patient who is symptomatic, or requires even routine diagnostic laboratory work, may be hospitalized. Physicians' offices have ceased to be places of treatment, and have become merely clearing houses where the well are separated from the sick, who are sent to the hospital to see if they are sick enough to be in the hospital. . . . This is an easy way to practice medicine, and as long as there is an insurance company, Blue Cross, or the Fund to pick up the tab, everyone is happy.[51]

Charleston area administrators noted that this problem also became more prevalent as the size of the beneficiary pool decreased. As the number of paying patients fell, hospitals were tempted to increase the length-of-stay of those that continued to be covered in order to keep beds full.[52] AMO review provided only imperfect safeguards against this behavior.

In addition to the lack of appropriate facilities, the Fund's attempt to reduce its reliance on hospitalization was hampered by the lack, in some regions, of an adequate supply of physicians sympathetic to the Fund. The AMOs' attempts to encourage physicians to provide care in the most cost-effective manner were less successful in areas where physicians resisted Fund review. This situation forced administrators like those at Johnstown to conclude, "It is becoming increasingly apparent that the present method of dealing only with individual physicians whom we know are essential and necessary to provide medical service to our patient group is the most effective approach yet devised to insure high quality care at reasonable cost."[53] Thus the underdevelopment of the full range of health care facilities in the mining regions combined with instances of excess hospital capacity and insufficient numbers of physicians willing to control costs further augmented the tendency toward excessive reliance upon hospital care already inherent in the Fund's program.

Second, the Fund's beneficiaries possessed a number of characteristics that also led them to rely heavily on specialist and hospital care. In general, Fund beneficiaries could be expected to make greater use of the health care system as compared to the general population due to, in the words of Warren Draper, "a number of reasons centering largely around the sociological difference between the Fund population and the general population."[54] More specifically, the age profile of the beneficiary pool was particularly responsible for higher utilization rates, "Since utilization of medical services is greater in the older unemployed persons, we may anticipate a relatively higher rate of services for awhile until the backlog of remedial conditions have been removed. Medical conditions most commonly found in this group seems to be arthritis in some form, cardiovascular disease and pulmonary dysfunction."[55]

The relatively low education levels of beneficiaries also resulted in excessive use of health care. For example, in 1955 the Birmingham AMO completed a study of patients who had been hospitalized 20 or more times in the previous five years. These high hospitalization rates were not a result, by and large, of inaccurate diagnoses but, rather, poor patient understanding of their diagnoses and treatment regimens.[56]

Furthermore, living in remote communities, the health of Fund beneficiaries was adversely affected by poor living standards, inadequate sanitation, and the absence of public health programs. The difficulty of transportation to adequate medical facilities often forced beneficiaries to postpone seeking treatment until specialist or hospital care was required. Finally, miners were exposed to significant occupational hazards which increased their demands for specialized care. All of these factors produce high utilization of hospitals, regardless of the absence or presence of coverage for routine care.

Fund administrators had various tools to correct for the program's bias toward specialist and hospital care at the expense of primary care. The most excessive and inappropriate cases of utilization could be corrected through the usual channels of AMO review. More systematic instances of overutilization were addressed by the managed care initiatives that will be discussed in chapters 4 and 5: the participating physicians list, the managing physician concept, and retainer payments. The evaluation of these programs demonstrates the difficulties the Fund encountered in attempting to accommodate its tendency to promote specialist and hospital care, given the difficulties posed by the characteristics of the mining regions and populations.

CHAPTER FOUR

The Delivery of Physician Care under the Fund's Managed Care Initiatives

*T*he set of managed care policies administrators devised to modify providers' behavior constituted the Fund's greatest deviation from mainstream medical care. In an attempt to reduce costs, the Fund sought to decrease reliance on hospitalization, to reduce unnecessary surgery and treatment procedures, and to increase preventive care. Simultaneously, the Fund strove to increase the quality of care that beneficiaries received. Administrators attempted to weave together their dual objectives of making care cost-effective while enhancing its quality in the managed care policies that they aimed at providers. This was a difficult task given that improvements in the quality of care tend to also increase the demand for care. The resultant higher costs necessitated further controls aimed at curbing excessive utilization.

This chapter will focus on the Fund's attempts to influence the cost and quality of physician care. The Fund's major initiatives in this realm were the establishment of a panel of participating physicians, the assignment of a managing physician to each beneficiary, and the organization of group practices. The Fund also sought to influence physician behavior by moving away from fee-for-service reimbursement toward retainer, or fee-for-time payments for physician care.

Because Fund policies deviated so radically from established patterns of relations between payers and providers, they required constant monitoring and coordination. Fund administrators chose to implement the policies aimed at altering provider behavior gradually, paying close attention to developing initiatives that reinforced one another as part of an overall package. The pace of reform also was dictated by the level of development of the coalfields' medical infrastructure. Unwilling to be constrained constantly by substandard physicians and hospitals, the Fund sponsored many initiatives to boost the quality of the infrastructure.

The Fund would eventually go so far as to build and operate its own set of hospitals in the late 1950s and early 1960s. Relatively more attention has been paid to the Fund's hospitals as the most visible component of its programs and a discussion of the hospital chain will be reserved for the next chapter. While the reforms outlined and evaluated here may not have received as much attention as the hospitals, they were nevertheless as radical and probably did more to achieve the Fund's objectives of increasing the quality of care while ensuring that the cost-effectiveness of the delivery of care was maximized. The initiatives that the Fund sponsored resemble closely the underlying tenets of modern health maintenance organizations (HMOs). Predating the widespread application of HMOs by three decades and caring for a beneficiary population with demanding health needs, the Fund's experience offers a unique opportunity to test the effectiveness of managed care policies.

The Participating Physician List

The Fund's first major concern in improving physician care was to increase the supply of qualified physicians available to its beneficiaries. Due to the pressure to replace the company doctor system quickly, the Fund had little choice at the outset but to recruit local physicians to care for its clients. Persistent physician shortages and the continuing substandard level of physician care eventually induced administrators to recruit physicians from outside of the coalfields. While the Fund could not afford to pay much attention to the quality of those local physicians, administrators did show great concern for quality in recruiting outside physicians.

The administrators' first task in installing the Fund was to replace the reimbursement system for specialist and hospital care that had existed under the check-off plans. Providers would now receive payment for services from the Fund instead of from individual operators. Administrators at Area Medical Offices wrote to local physicians asking them to participate in this new arrangement. Lists of participating providers were then compiled and distributed to local unions so they could direct beneficiaries to these physicians. The lists were also used by physicians when making referrals. At its inception, the list was simply a directory of providers who agreed to bill the Fund for services rendered.

The infusion of funds for medical care made possible by the Fund attracted physicians to the coalfields. The Area Medical Administrator at the Louisville AMO noted, "Medical care has been literally pulled up by its bootstraps, as the economy of the East Kentucky counties would never have attracted well trained young physicians without the aid of the Welfare Fund."[1] As an example, the prospect of Fund reimbursement had attracted a board-certified thoracic surgeon, urologist, orthopedic surgeon, general surgeon, and a board-qualified internist to practice in Pikeville, Kentucky.[2] The Fund also recruited committed young doctors from the U.S. Public Health Service, the Farm Security Agency, and the National Health Service Corps to work in areas of the coalfields that lacked qualified physicians. Significantly, the Fund searched for physicians who shared its managed care philosophy. These progressive physicians reported abuses of the medical care system,[3] and eventually helped ease the implementation of reforms.

Over time, the Fund altered the participating physician list so that it came to resemble a closed panel and not just a list of doctors willing to bill the Fund. Explaining the rationale for this change, Draper noted, "I think that free choice of physicians should be limited to physicians who are willing to conserve the resources of the paying agency to the fullest extent possible."[4] As a first step, the Fund established three basic criteria that physicians were required to meet for inclusion in the list: they agreed to bill the Fund directly and accept its reimbursement as full payment for services; they agreed to refrain from submitting excessive charges and prescribing excessive treatment; and they agreed to perform only those services for which they were certified. Under the first requirement, the Fund did not allow participating physicians to charge beneficiaries copayments or deductibles.[5] This requirement prevented physicians from simply passing on to beneficiaries charges above those deemed reasonable by the Fund.

Second, participating physicians agreed not to engage in the abuses— excessive charges, charges for work not performed, and the prescription of unnecessary treatment—that the Fund sought to eradicate. Administrators built relationships with providers so that suspected abuses could be corrected through correspondence and discussion. For instance, when the Fund discovered that physicians at a particular hospital delivered 19 percent of babies by cesarean section, administrators at the local AMO initiated a series of discussions with the hospital to further educate the hospital's physicians. As a result, the hospital's cesarean rate dropped to just 2 percent of all deliveries.[6] The Fund did not limit itself to critiquing individual providers when problems were more broad-based. For instance, in 1954, Johnstown AMO administrators concerned over the high level of hospital admissions and the long lengths-of-stay in area hospitals began discussions with local medical societies, engaged in discussions with individual physicians, circulated detailed studies of services provided by the Fund to hospital staffs, and sent a letter to all area participating physicians outlining sources of overutilization of hospital resources the AMO had identified.[7]

When providers did not respond to these attempts by the AMO to curb unreasonable practices, the AMOs could remove them from the list. For example, the Johnstown AMO removed from the list two physicians found guilty of ghost surgery and fee-splitting.[8] Eliminating unacceptable providers from the list also affected the behavior of providers who remained on the list. For instance, the Birmingham AMO noted that its discontinuation of a teaching hospital at the Medical College of Alabama sent a signal to other local hospitals about the need to pay close attention to costs and utilization.[9]

Simply threatening removal from the list sometimes provided the desired change in behavior, as an area medical administrator noted, "The Area office in its public relations efforts has had some effect, yet we must admit readily that the most potent public relations instrument we have had, has been the authority to authorize payment."[10] For instance, when the Louisville AMO threatened to take to Protestant Deaconess Hospital off its list as a result of the hospital's high cost of care, the hospital reduced its drug prices by 20 percent across-the-board.[11] This threat was particularly potent where the Fund had alternatives to suspect providers. The Morgantown AMO, for example, did not have any success in improving conditions at Brownsville General Hospital until the opening of the Centerville Clinic. Faced with competition from the ambulatory care available at Centerville, the Brownsville Board of Trustees agreed to enter into discussions with the AMO concerning improvements in its services and charges, and furthermore, granted Centerville physicians admitting privileges.[12]

Third, the Fund insisted that participating physicians possess qualifications for the procedures they performed.[13] This requirement was directed primarily at physicians performing surgical procedures as, especially in the Fund's initial period of operation, most surgery was performed by general practitioners. In 1953, a Fund report found that general practitioners' rates of surgery were excessive and recommended that only members of the American College of Surgeons or doctors certified by the American Board of Surgery be allowed to operate. This initiative was intended both to protect beneficiaries from receiving substandard care and to decrease the costs associated with excessive rates of surgery. The Fund claimed that this policy resulted in an immediate two-thirds decrease in hospital admissions for surgery.[14]

Fund administrators found it comparatively easy to ensure that participating physicians accepted payments in full from the Fund and bore the requisite qualifications. However, requiring providers to refrain from providing excessive care and from submitting excessive charges proved more difficult to enforce. Not only did asymmetries of information between the Fund and the providers make it difficult to detect abuses but, once detected, abuses were difficult to reverse in instances where physicians proved to be uncooperative. Given the shortage of physicians in the coalfields and the Fund's desire to build harmonious relations with local medical societies, in its early years the Fund could not afford to eliminate from the list all physicians suspected of prescribing unnecessary treatment or submitting excessive charges. Thus, instead of using the list as a means of preventing certain physicians from providing services to beneficiaries, the Fund initially used the participating physician list as a tool to educate physicians.

For most of the 1950s, the Fund used the participating physician list to impart to providers its insistence on close attention to costs and appropriate treatment. The Fund's administrators hoped to persuade physicians to work with their corresponding AMO and to accept its counsel when their charges or treatments differed markedly from local norms. In addition, the AMOs and the Fund's national office attempted to persuade medical societies to heighten their monitoring of members and their censure of those found to be in violation of medical ethics codes. Emphasizing physician education and the cultivation of relationships with local medical societies, the Fund refrained from eliminating all but the most abusive physicians from the list during the early 1950s.

After seven years of experience with the participating physicians list, however, Fund administrators concluded that their attempts to educate individual physicians and to work with organized medicine had not achieved the desired increase in quality of care and reduction in costs. The Fund shifted its approach and instituted policy changes that hastened the transformation of the participating physician list into a policy that more closely resembled a closed panel. In 1957 Warren Draper issued a directive to all AMO administrators mandating deep cuts in the list of participating physicians.[15] Lists were to be pared down to include only those providers that administrators were completely confident provided satisfactory service. As a result, almost a third of the physicians were removed from the list. Most of the physicians who were dropped had been singled out for prescribing unnecessary treatment or submitting excessive charges, and had been proven to be unwilling to alter their behavior. In addition, a minority of physicians who provided only a small amount of service to Fund beneficiaries were dropped from the list in order to economize on administrative costs.

The Fund's review of this rather drastic and sudden policy change confirmed the administrators' conjecture that despite its efforts to educate physicians, excesses had continued to exist under the previous policy regime. The Fund reported that in the ten months following the policy change, one state's hospital admissions decreased by 11.6 percent, surgical operations fell by 14.4 percent, and total costs decreased by 7.5 percent. The Fund claimed that this policy shift reduced expenses by almost a million dollars in the following fiscal year.[16] While the 1957 directive did reduce utilization and costs in the following year, the gains from the restricted participating physicians list proved to be transitory. A closer examination of the administrators' expectations and the effect of the cut helps explain why the gains were not sustainable.

Draper expected a number of benefits to result from narrowing the list of participating physicians. First, monitoring would become more efficient and more effective as fewer physicians served greater numbers of beneficiaries. Second, as positions on the list became scarce, physicians would have greater incentives to "screen their patients for hospitalization more carefully, avoid unnecessary x-ray and laboratory procedures, and make a special effort to please the patient and the Fund by rendering the best quality of service they can." Third, reductions in the number of available physicians would reduce "doctor shopping" by beneficiaries. Finally, decreasing the number of hospitals on the list would lower the number of vacant beds and, consequently, the probability that beneficiaries would be hospitalized simply in order to help cover the costs of hospital operations.[17]

Draper's directive was not a departure from Fund practices, but served to accelerate trimming of the participating physicians list already in progress. In fact, many administrators welcomed the directive's catalyzing effect and seemed particularly grateful that the unprecedented level of cuts would be seen as part of general Fund policy and not simply as the isolated actions of local administrators.[18] Charleston administrators, for example, stated that the cuts, "provided the vehicle for a much sounder approach to our multitudinous problems than has possibly any single directive provided the Area Medical Administrators for a long, long time. . . . We call the present program 'Operation Rat-hole.' It is designed to provide a defense against the abuse of Fund resources by some physicians, hospitals, community agencies, and beneficiaries."[19] Overall, approximately 29 percent of physicians were removed from the Fund's participating physicians list. Cuts were particularly deep in the Morgantown and Johnstown areas. The Morgantown AMO terminated the use of 45 percent of its 466 participating physicians, removed 12 hospitals from its list, and restricted the use of five of the remaining 17 hospitals on its list.[20] Johnstown reduced its participating physicians list by two-thirds.[21]

Administrators unanimously concluded that the 1957 cut reduced excessive utilization of services and thereby rendered cost savings. An examination of hospital admission rates, surgery rates, and expenditures per beneficiary in the year following the cut reveals that administrators were correct as far as the short-term decrease in utilization was concerned. However, there is no data to evaluate their claim that only excessive and unnecessary utilization was decreased. The AMOs' ability to monitor and review physician behavior would have provided some security that this reduction was restricted to unnecessary utilization. More importantly, however, further analysis shows that the gains from the reduction of the participating physicians list did not accrue beyond 1958.

The overall Fund admission rates decreased by 11.6 percent from 1957 to 1958, by far the largest annual decrease in the admission rate for the entire period studied (see Table 7). Among the individual areas, the Louisville, Charleston, Beckley, and Johnstown AMOs registered the largest decreases in admission rates. The overall Fund surgery rate decreased by 6.6 percent in the year after the cut, registering the second largest annual decrease in the period for which these data were collected (1952–66). All areas except Denver experienced declines in surgery rates with the largest decreases occurring in Morgantown, Birmingham, and St. Louis.[22] Finally, the overall expenditure per beneficiary increased a mere 0.1 percent from 1957 to 1958, the smallest increase in the period prior to 1965 and far less than the 8.3 percent increase registered in the previous year.[23] Expenditures per beneficiary actually fell in Louisville, Birmingham, Charleston, and Morgantown.[24]

The magnitude of these declines in admission rates, surgery rates, and expenditures per beneficiary suggests that the 1957 participating physicians list cut, as the only major policy change of that year, was primarily responsible for halting or reversing the upward trends in these variables. However, it is equally true that the reversions to trend by 1959 suggest that the effect of the 1957 cut was only temporary. By 1959, all AMOs, with the exception of Denver, registered increases in their admission rates; all areas experienced increases in surgery rates and in expenditures per beneficiary.[25]

It is difficult to determine why the benefits from the 1957 cut that were so evident in 1958 largely disappeared by 1959. Some administrators appeared to realize at the time of the cut that the potential for gains might

Table 7   Percentage change in hospital admissions per 1,000 beneficiaries, surgeries per 1,000 beneficiaries, and expenditures per beneficiary in the year following the 1957 participating physicians list reduction

	Percentage Change from 1957 to 1958		
	Admissions	Surgeries	Expenditure
Louisville	−16.2%	−5.2%	−3.0%
Charleston	−13.6	−8.4	−1.9
Beckley	−13.4	−2.4	0.2
Johnstown	−12.2	−5.6	1.3
Birmingham	−11.3	−10.5	−2.6
Denver	−10.3	10.5	5.2
Knoxville	−9.8	−7.1	2.9
Morgantown	−9.5	−13.0	−1.5
Pittsburgh	−6.8	−5.5	2.5
St. Louis	−3.3	−10.4	1.5
All Areas	−11.6%	−6.6%	0.1%

Sources: Rates of admission and surgery are in UMWA Office of Research and Statistics, "Statistical Reports," various years, Fund Archives; expenditure per beneficiary are in UMWA Executive Medical Officer, "Subject Files," various years, Fund Archives.

only be transitory. Johnstown administrators noted that while the cut was responsible for an "immediate decrease in our hospital admission rates," one of the "two most important questions [was] how long this reaction would last."[26] Morgantown administrators went further and noted that the 1957 cut was unlikely to be a panacea for high costs and excessive utilization:

> We believe that further efforts to reduce costs by eliminating more physicians and hospitals in the Morgantown Area will show diminishing returns. Until better organization for the provision of medical care is provided through increased availability of good quality ambulatory patient care and specialists services through the media of group practice clinics, we will have to do the best we can with the best qualified physicians available.[27]

With their penchant for viewing the Fund's programs as an integrated whole, administrators placed little faith in the ability of individual policy modifications to produce sweeping changes. In addition the Fund's trustees, concerned with the overall operating budget of the Fund, were also soon aware that the cut in the participating physicians list would not stop the Fund's slide into operating deficits in 1958, 1959, and 1960 (see chapter 6).

The Fund's decision to transform the participating physicians list into a closed panel had other consequences besides reducing costs. First, the Fund did not endear itself to organized medicine by alleging that a large number of physicians were engaging in suspect treatment and billing practices and then preventing these physicians from caring for Fund beneficiaries. However, by the late 1950s Fund administrators doubted whether relations between the Fund and many local medical societies would ever be harmonious given the Fund's adherence to managed care practices (see chapter 6). Hence, increasing the ire of already uncooperative medical societies appeared to involve only relatively minor costs to the Fund.

Second, reducing the size of the list also restricted the choice of physicians available to Fund beneficiaries. While the extent of this restriction on the local level is unclear, overall a number of factors compensated for the cost to beneficiaries of this restriction. For instance, by the late 1950s, the Fund had succeeded in recruiting a significant number of qualified physicians to the coalfields so that the physicians that remained on the list were more likely to be those capable of providing high caliber service. Furthermore, beneficiaries benefited from the removal of physicians who prescribed costly, and possibly harmful, excessive treatment. Finally, it can be argued that since the Fund was self-insured, the cost savings from this policy change ultimately accrued to beneficiaries, and thereby offset to some degree the cost of restricting their choice of physicians.

The participating physician list was the Fund's first attempt to address the asymmetries of information that exist between the payer and the provider of medical care. By accepting into the plan only providers who had a proven track record of prescribing and charging for treatment in a reasonable fashion, the AMO reduced the potential of excessive utilization and charges. The list did not eliminate every instance of excess, but it did serve to create a pool of physicians who, in principle, adhered to the Fund's philosophy of providing cost-effective care. The selection of these physicians was critical in that it enabled the Fund to implement more ambitious reforms of physician care.

The Managing Physician

While the participating physician list went some distance toward ensuring that beneficiaries visited only physicians who conformed to the Fund's payment or treatment standards, it did not limit the number of participating doctors from whom the clients could seek treatment. Some beneficiaries responded to this unrestricted access to providers by overutilizing the services of costly specialists and hospitals. Moreover, since the Fund did not control beneficiaries' access to and use of primary care—still commonly handled through check-off plans—it had no way of controlling referrals from primary care physicians to specialists on the list.

For example, an area medical administrator examining the hospitalization experiences of 2,845 beneficiaries over four years discovered that 18 had been admitted an average of 28 times and that one beneficiary had been admitted an staggering 83 times. The 17 physicians involved in admitting these patients had communicated little among themselves in the course of prescribing treatment. In addition, the possibility that the patients themselves might be able to coordinate the physicians' efforts was low given that the physicians lacked the time to explain fully the diagnosis and prescribed therapeutic regimen to the patients.[28]

As a complement to the participating physician list, the Fund attempted to assign each beneficiary to a single physician, known as a managing physician, on the list. The managing physician acted as a "gatekeeper" by approving visits to other specialists or hospitals, thereby decreasing the potential for unnecessary visits to other providers. In addition, the continuity of care afforded by this arrangement increased the probability that an appropriate diagnosis would be made. Better diagnoses would reduce the drain on the Fund's resources fostered by unnecessary hospitalization and specialist visits. Moreover, the Fund selected internists to act as managing physicians as these physicians did not face incentives to perform surgery themselves, thereby further reducing the potential for unnecessary hospitalization.[29]

Managing physicians were particularly effective in handling beneficiaries who entered the hospital frequently. As part of a 1956 pilot program, the Birmingham AMO assigned three managing physicians working in one group practice to care for 300 multiple admission cases.[30] The managing physicians spent generous amounts of time examining each patient, determining a diagnosis, and explaining the diagnosis to the patient. Reviewing the experience of the first 76 patients placed in the program between January 1956 and April 1958, the AMO found that the group's annual admission rate fell 44 percent, from 2.3 admissions per year before enrollment in the program to 1.3 admissions per year after assignment to a managing physician. This generated a $51,238 savings over the 20-month period studied, or an average of $375 in annual savings per patient.[31]

The continuity of care fostered by the managing physician arrangement also was intended to increase early detection and prevention of illness. Since illnesses are typically less expensive and less painful to treat in early stages of development, early detection and prevention should have reduced the

Fund's outlays and increased beneficiaries' well-being. It is difficult to evaluate how successful managing physicians were in this regard. While continuity of care probably does increase the chances that a physician will detect an illness early and engage in preventive medicine, it is unlikely that continuity of care, by itself, ensures that maximum attention to these practices occurred. Most notably, early detection is dependent upon the patient's timely visit to the physician's office. Moreover, it is unclear how these managing physicians interacted with primary care physicians, most of whom practiced outside of Fund control. Group practices offered the highest probability of coordination of these efforts (see below) with the result that attention to preventive care was more likely to occur in these settings.

In summary, the assignment of managing physicians to Fund beneficiaries was designed to overcome the bias toward specialist and hospital care inherent in the program by limiting beneficiaries' access to this costly care. The Fund placed the decision to use these services in the hands of physicians who not only had the requisite medical knowledge to prescribe such care, but who also treated beneficiaries on an ongoing basis. The Fund's hopes that this arrangement would increase the practice of preventive medicine by increasing the continuity of care is more difficult to evaluate given the Fund's lack of coverage for primary care. It is likely that managing physicians were best able to achieve the Fund's dual objectives of decreasing the costs of medical care and increasing the quality of care received by chronic users of care by treating them in group practice settings.

Group Practices

The Fund's efforts to help organize and finance group practices represented a far more explicit attempt than the policies aimed at individual physicians to control costs and improve the quality of care available to beneficiaries. Increases in the quality of care derived primarily from the enhanced range of services that group practices could provide. Cost savings resulted from the greater coordination and review of care that occurred when physicians worked together as a unit. Group practices were also better able to avoid unnecessary hospitalization and specialist care by providing more comprehensive services.[32] For example, providing extensive outpatient services acted as a lower cost substitute for hospitalization.[33]

In its first two decades, the Fund helped develop between 30 and 50 group practice clinics located primarily in central Appalachia (see Table 8, Map 2).[34] It is important to note that in developing group practices, the Fund once again was promoting a system of care that deviated significantly from established relations between beneficiaries, providers, and payers. Its efforts were pioneering as group practice was still a novelty during this period. In 1951 there were only 459 listed group practices in the United States, employing only 2 to 3 percent of all physicians.[35] By 1959, the number of group practices had more than tripled to 1,546, but the proportion of physicians working in group practices still comprised only 7.1 percent of all physicians.[36] Thus, the Fund's efforts came at a time when group practices were growing in popularity but still included the services of only a small number of physicians.

Group practices in the coalfields typically were organized as a cluster of clinics. A main clinic employing 10 to 30 physicians would be established in regions that had the requisite density of beneficiaries to support the clinic. To serve outlying communities, the main clinic would establish one to three smaller branch offices employing two to four physicians each.[37] Group practices were most useful to the Fund where a significant number of beneficiaries lived in close proximity to the clinics.

The Fund helped stimulate the development of group practices in regions that either lacked physicians or that lacked physicians sympathetic to the Fund's practices.[38] For instance, the Fund established group practices in the West Virginia towns of Oceana and Smithers where physician care had been practically unavailable. Similarly, larger group practices like those in Fairmont, West Virginia, and Bellaire, Ohio, established branch offices to serve outlying areas that otherwise were underserved.[39] The Fund also promoted the formation of group practices in regions where local physicians were "antagonistic"[40] to the Fund and its policies: the Jefferson Health Foundation in Birmingham, Alabama; the Daniel Boone Clinic in Harlan, Kentucky; and the clinics in New Kensington and Fairmont, Pennsylvania, were all opened as alternatives to established providers.

The Fund's role in the emergence of group practices consisted of aiding in the establishment of clinics and acting as a major payer once the clinics began operations. The establishment of the Russellton Clinic has been particularly well-studied and serves to illustrate the role of the Fund in developing group practices.[41] In 1952 local union officials approached the Pittsburgh AMO for help in hiring a new check-off doctor to replace a departing physician.[42] The AMO viewed this request with particular urgency as it sought to avoid the increase in hospitalization that typically resulted when a community was without a physician.

Through its efforts to recruit physicians to underdeveloped areas like Russellton, AMO administrators found that it was easier to attract doctors to group than to solo practices. In addition, even at this early stage, the

Table 8 Group Practices serving Fund beneficiaries

Medical Group	Offices	Location
Jefferson Medical Group	Jefferson Medical Group	Birmingham,AL
	Jackson Clinic	Jasper, AL
	Adamsville Clinic	Adamsville, AL
	Bessemer Clinic	Bessemer, AL
Cumberland Medical Group	Cumberland Clinic	Cumberland, KY
	Lynch Medical Services	Lynch, KY
Centerville Medical Group	Centerville Clinic	Centerville, PA
	Carmichaels Clinic	Carmichaels, PA
	California Community Office	California, PA
	Vestaburg Community Office	Vestaburg, PA
	Marianna Community Office	Marianna, PA
Russellton Medical Group	Russellton Clinic	Russellton, PA
	New Kensington Clinic	New Kensington, PA
	Acmetonia Community Office	Acmetonia, PA
	Apollo Community Office	Apollo, PA
	Sharon Medical Clinic	Sharon, PA
Bellaire Medical Group	Bellaire Clinic	Bellaire, OH
	Harrisville Clinic	Harrisville, OH
	Community Clinic of Powhatan	Powhatan, OH
Clear Fork Medical Group	Oceana Medical Center	Oceana, WV
Longacre Medical Group	Longacre Medical Center	Longacre, WV
	Cedar Grove Community Office	Cedar Grove, WV
Raleigh–Boone Medical Group	Raleigh–Boone Medical Center	Whitesville, WV
	Montcoal Community Office	Montcoal, WV
Fairmont Medical Group	Fairmont Clinic	Fairmont, WV
	Grant Town Community Office	Grant Town, WV
	Farmington Community Office	Farmington, WV
	Shinnston Community Office	Shinnston, WV
Laird Foundation	Summersville Clinic and Hospital	Summersville, WV
N.A.	Golden Clinic Memorial Hospital	Elkins, WV
N.A.	Myers Clinic	Philippi, WV
N.A.	N.A.	Palmer, TN
N.A.	Richlands Clinic	Richlands, VA
		Clinch, VA
		Mattie, VA
N.A.	Grundy Clinic	Grundy, VA
N.A.	Dickenson County Clinic	Clintwood, VA
N.A.	Springfield Clinic	Springfield, IL
N.A.	Carbondale Clinic	Carbondale, IL
Utah Permanente Hospital	Dragerton Medical Care Plan	Dragerton, UT

Sources: Leslie Falk, "Group Health Plans in Coal Mining Communities," *Journal of Health and Human Behavior* 4 (Spring 1963); American Labor Health Association, "Group Practice Medical Care Plans Providing Services to Labor Groups," 1958, Lorin Edgar Kerr Papers; UMWA Welfare and Retirement Fund, Area Medical Offices, "Information Reports," various years, Fund Archives.

Map 2 Location of group practices serving Fund beneficiaries

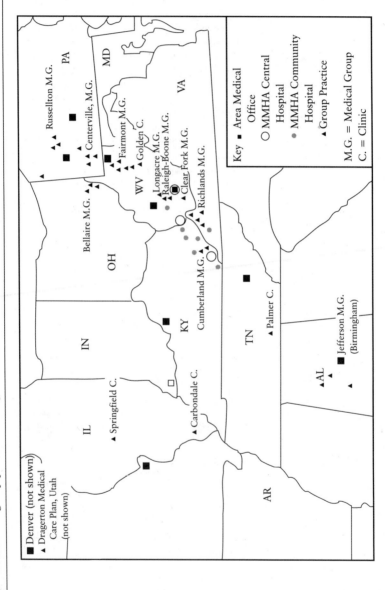

Fund's administrators were convinced that group practices were superior to solo practitioners. The Fund, therefore, decided that it would help create a group practice in Russellton rather than simply recruit an individual general practitioner to serve the area's beneficiaries. The Fund induced a local general practitioner to search for other doctors with whom he could establish a group practice by assuring him that the Fund would include the resulting practice on its participating physician list. In addition, the Fund instructed the local that had submitted the request for the physician to find other locals willing to use the new group practice in order to build the patient base necessary to support the clinic. The petitioning local found two other locals with which it formed a nonprofit corporation—the governing board—which raised funds for the construction of the clinic, and eventually owned and operated the facilities. In addition, the board also arranged a check-off plan to cover routine home and office care. Once the clinic began operations, the Fund reimbursed the physicians for the specialist and hospital services they provided on a retainer basis (see below).

The Fund's practice of stimulating the development of group practices became a mainstay of the AMOs' duties. For example in 1967, almost two decades after the creation of the Russellton group practice, the Fund helped establish the Oakwood Clinic to meet the demand for physicians that arose when mining expanded into new territories in western Virginia.[43] The Fund continued to aid in the evolution of established group practices by advocating the expansion of services to include home care programs, benefits counseling, and prepaid pharmaceutical services; by encouraging increases in research and educational activities; and by approaching other groups in the communities to join the clinics.[44]

The group practices that the Fund helped establish were also notable for their unique administrative structure.[45] In particular, the Fund designed the group practices to include an unprecedented degree of community participation in the overall operation of the clinics. To begin with, the clinics were not owned by the physicians but, rather, by nonprofit governing boards comprised of members of the local community. The boards rented the facilities to the physicians who, in turn, agreed not to own or operate medical facilities or major equipment in their area of operation. The boards also determined the general policies of the clinics.

The physicians' role in group practices was largely limited to providing medical services subject to oversight by the governing boards and the Fund. Each clinic's physicians were led by a medical director chosen by the physicians and approved by the clinic's governing board. The medical director was ultimately responsible to both the physicians and the board. Any additional physicians selected by the clinic's physicians to join the practice had to be approved by the clinic's board and by the Fund.[46]

The composition of the governing boards varied by clinic. For example, the Russellton Clinic's board was comprised solely of UMWA officials (15 local officials and two district officials) while the Bellaire Clinic's governing board included a Steelworkers' Union official and six community professionals in addition to 10 UMWA officials.[47] It is important to realize that the ability of the governing board to have meaningful input into the policies of the clinic often was circumscribed by asymmetries of information that made it difficult for board members to dictate medical policies to physicians. As a result, Boyd has charged that the boards sometimes operated as a "passive, elite" group.[48] Paradoxically, while the governing boards were intended to increase community participation in the provision of health care, it appears that the most active boards were those made up primarily of miners.[49] In fact, it may be more accurate to characterize the governing boards as venues for rank-and-file miners, instead of the "community" at large, to become involved in the operation of the clinics. Miners were particularly active as the boards were the only avenue they had to participate directly in decisions concerning their health benefits, albeit at a local level. Decisions regarding policy changes—including eligibility rules and benefit levels—were made by Fund administrators at the regional and national levels and were not discussed with the rank-and-file (see chapter 6).

The Fund helped create group practices not only to increase the supply of physicians, but also to increase the quality of health care providers available to beneficiaries. The Fund designed group practices to provide a wider array of services than could be provided by an individual physician. Moreover, care was supplied in a setting that promoted the Fund's practice of continual review in order to increase the probability of accurate diagnoses and appropriate treatment.[50]

First, group practices provided comprehensive care by supplying the greatest possible range of services from routine care to multispecialty care.[51] Unlike solo physicians, group practices enjoyed the resources and patient base necessary to employ auxiliary personnel and specialists. Fund administrators stressed, however, that group practices not function as "mere aggregations of specialists," but rather that they "develop systematic cooperation" between all clinic employees.[52]

Auxiliary personnel—including physical therapists, podiatrists, optometrists, psychologists, social workers, and inhalation therapists— performed some of the functions the group's physicians would have to do if in solo practice, thereby reserving the physicians' time for those functions only they could perform. In fact, the specialized training and experience of auxiliary personnel often enabled them to provide better services than physicians.[53]

The use of specialists enabled the clinic to augment its range of services. Due to the scarce supply of specialists in the coalfields, the Fund often used its close links to the group practices to improve the allocation of their services. For example, the Charleston AMO helped the Delbarton Highlands Clinic arrange for different specialists—in medicine, pediatrics, surgery, obstetrics, and family planning—to visit on different days of the week.[54] As a result of the employment of auxiliary personnel and specialists in an integrated fashion, group practices realized cost savings while expanding their range of services.[55]

The enhanced range of care offered by the group practices was appreciated not only by the beneficiaries, but also by the physicians themselves. Instead of practicing as solo practitioners in isolated areas, physicians working in group practices retained closer contact with colleagues and with advances in medical treatment. These advantages became a potent recruiting device in enlisting physicians for practice in the coalfields.

Second, in addition to being comprehensive, the care provided by group practices was also coordinated. Physicians employed in the group practices operated as a unit, engaging in managed care, peer review, and continuing education to enhance the quality of care that beneficiaries received. Consistent with the policies outlined above, each beneficiary was assigned to a managing physician, despite the availability of a number of physicians at any particular clinic. The number of physicians in a group practice ensured that the beneficiary would have some choice in selecting a physician, while the ultimate assignment to one managing physician ensured that the beneficiary did not receive redundant care.

Coordinated care also was achieved through peer review of diagnosis and treatment decisions. Essentially, this practice augmented the AMOs' review of providers' services by encouraging physicians in group practices to scrutinize each other's decisions in order to reduce unnecessary care.[56] As one group physician explained, "No doctor can afford to practice shabby medicine in this clinic, where he is always under the scrutiny of his associates and the residents. If he should do anything wrong, he knows he can be asked what he did, how he did it and why he did it. It's not like being spied on; it's a stimulus, a constant challenge to keep your standards high."[57]

Third, group practices were more likely than solo practitioners to promote continuing physician education. In part, this result is inherent in the nature of group practice as physicians are in constant contact with colleagues who have different types of training and levels of experience. Most group practices in the coalfields, moreover, explicitly mandated ongoing education of their members. For example, the Russellton Clinic required its members to devote one half-day a week to their education and to spend one two-week period a year at conferences or seminars.[58] The Fund also encouraged group practices to take advantage of their size and unique composition to forge ties with research institutions; for example, the clinics at Centerville, Russellton, and Bellaire all established links with the University of Pittsburgh.[59]

Finally, all three policies—managing physicians, peer review, and education —should also have served to reinforce group physicians' attention to preventive medicine.[60] However, without Fund reimbursement for primary care, attention to preventive care was limited. A Fund administrator surveying group practices in Pennsylvania noted, "Although interest in preventive medicine was well demonstrated . . . and although opportunities for specially organized preventive services are far greater in prepaid group practice than in private solo practice, little real progress has been made in this area."[61] Preventive medicine occurred primarily in the form of classes for diabetics, well-baby and prenatal care programs, and largely overlooked the "apparently healthy."[62]

The quality of care supplied by group practices exceeded that available through most solo practitioners in the coalfields. Reviewing the experience of the Centerville Clinic in 1970, two Fund administrators reflected,

> Centerville, like certain other Fund-related clinics, exists in a world apart from traditional medical practice. Here, through years of effort and influence, we have shaped a model for miners with which there is little to compare in the ordinary universe of medical care. . . . a picture of a patient in a rural community, seen promptly, especially in emergencies; with general physicians, specialists and ancillary personnel of every description at hand, including mental health workers; receiving modern diagnostic services such as laboratory, x-ray, electrocardiogram, and many other procedures . . . When confused or unable to understand health problems, as is the case frequently with all patients, miners receive advice from receptionists and specialists such as social workers, registered nurses and counselors of various kinds. When they leave, they take medicines with them; when they need it, they receive home visits . . . To top it all, this clinic

belongs to and is operated by representatives of the major consumers themselves—the miners; not by physicians, or the Fund, or government . . . This program is the goal of labor and many other consumer groups and its costs, therefore, cannot be measured in terms of the usual busy doctor's office where weeks are required for an appointment, lengthy waiting upon arrival is the rule, and visits to other offices or the hospital are required to complete the diagnosis and to begin therapy.[63]

The comprehensive and coordinated nature of group practice care not only enhanced quality of care, but also delivered cost savings to the Fund. Group practices enabled physicians to share equipment, thereby reducing the proliferation of underutilized equipment in individual practitioners' offices. The range of services provided by group practices also attracted a wider patient base than did those of solo practitioners. This enabled group practices to spread their costs over a patient pool that included the non-mining population, and to increase the likelihood of receiving support from government agencies.[64] Occasionally the Fund made explicit efforts to recruit other groups in the communities—such as steelworkers, farmers, and even students—to use the group practices.[65]

Finally, group practices also were expected to render cost savings in the form of lower hospitalization rates.[66] Leslie Falk maintained that in some areas, group practices lowered hospital admission rates by 25 percent.[67] Consistent with Falk's findings, the Russellton Clinic outside of Pittsburgh noted that its annual hospitalization rate of 75 to 80 beneficiaries per 1,000 was considerably lower than the rate of 125 beneficiaries per 1,000 in the area covered by the Pittsburgh AMO, and the rate of 160 beneficiaries per 1,000 for the Fund as a whole.[68] The Russellton group attributed its lower hospitalization rate to its "extensive diagnostic facilities, specialist participation, and roster of ancillary personnel."[69] The Pittsburgh AMO estimated that group practices in its area delivered savings of $200,000 to $300,000 in 1954.[70] Overall, group practices were a significant characteristic of the development of a region's medical care infrastructure. As such, their availability provided a substitute for more costly hospital care.[71]

One of the most interesting studies of the advantages of group practices was done in the Knoxville AMO in 1956.[72] The Knoxville area studied the experiences of two similar mining populations exposed to similar living conditions: one local union (1,148 miners and 7,090 beneficiaries) served by a group practice (Cumberland Valley Medical Group) in Lynch, Kentucky, and the other two local unions (950 miners and 4750 beneficiaries) served by general practitioners providing "inadequate classical 'camp doctor' care" in

Virginia.[73] Both populations had the option to purchase prepaid plans for services not covered by the Fund.[74] Beneficiaries in both populations were relatively young, employed by large operators, and were employed fully throughout the year. In addition, both populations had similar types of housing, sanitation, and public health facilities.

The Kentucky miners served by the group practice had a rate of hospitalization almost half that of the Virginia miners, largely due to the group practice's ability to treat patients in its outpatient clinic. While the Kentucky miners had longer lengths-of-stay once in the hospital, their rates of admission were still low enough to provide total hospital days that were below that of the Virginia miners.[75] The lower hospitalization rates also meant that the cost of hospitalization per person per year was considerably lower for the Kentucky group, despite the fact that day rates in the hospitals there were somewhat more expensive. The Fund spent roughly $51,000 per thousand beneficiaries in the Virginia locals and only $31,000 per thousand beneficiaries in the Kentucky locals.

The only significant drawback to group practices was their tendency to overemphasize specialist care. The St. Louis AMO noted,

> The chief trouble the Fund has in the use of [group practice] clinics is a tendency to over-serve and over-examine the patient with the result that the sweet wine of economy is spoiled and soured into the vinegar of extravagance. . . . The wise clinician does not need to perform every known laboratory and X-ray diagnostic service in order to recognize a psychoneurotic or hypochondriac patient.[76]

Pittsburgh area administrators noted that this distortion was not only typical, but expected given the Fund's reimbursement policies,

> The primary weakness of the program relates to a distortion common to most American clinic or group medical structures (and conditioned by the benefit policies of the UMWA Welfare Fund)—namely, the over-emphasis upon "central" specialist services and the converse starvation of the "peripheral" general or personal medical care.[77]

Overutilization was particularly likely to occur where group practices did not adequately integrate the services of general practitioners and, thus, functioned more as a collection of specialists practicing under one roof than as a coordinated team.

The Fund's development of group practices should not be viewed simply as another policy in its growing battery of managed care initiatives. Instead, group practices are better understood as part of the Fund's overall efforts to reform physician care. Group practices incorporated prior reforms into their operation and brought in-house the Fund's approach to cost-effective care. The environment that resulted provided the best conceivable set of opportunities for the physicians to achieve the Fund's objectives. Ironically, group practices also embodied the drawbacks present in a program designed to promote and control specialist care at the expense of primary care.

Prepayment of Services

The Fund reimbursed physicians for specialist and hospital care through either fee-for-service or retainer payments. Fee-for-service payments, the most common third-party payment method, reimbursed physicians for each treatment procedure performed. By contrast, retainer payments departed significantly from traditional reimbursement schemes by reimbursing physicians for the amount of time they devoted to caring for Fund beneficiaries.[78]

Retainer payments were designed to reduce the incentives for excessive and costly treatment inherent in the fee-for-service arrangement. Since the retainer mechanism does not reimburse providers separately for each surgical procedure, it removes the financial incentive to perform surgery where other, less costly treatments are available. Specifically, this payment method was designed to encourage physicians to spend the time necessary to accurately diagnose an ailment and prescribe an appropriate course of treatment. Moreover, retainer payments increased the ability of clinics in particular to provide preventive care,

> Since basic financing has been provided and the money barrier has been lessened, it is more feasible to offer the members health examinations; to interest them in immunizations, glaucoma screening, Pap smears, family planning; to reach them with a health newsletter, a family health conference, a multiphasic screening clinic, or psychosocial services. Major steps toward comprehensive care become possible.[79]

Given the low income level of residents of mining communities, it is unlikely that the clinics could have provided these services without retainer payments from the Fund.

It is important to stress that the Fund utilized retainer payments to complement the other practices described above—the participating physician list, managing physicians, and group practices—that also were designed to reduce unnecessary care. In particular, the Fund was an innovator in stimulating the development of prepaid group practice. While the number of group practices rose throughout the postwar period, the number of prepaid group practices remained relatively small throughout the 1950s and 1960s. In 1969 there were only 85 prepaid group practices in the United States.[80]

In addition, the Fund recognized that physicians often required more time to practice preventive care and to thoroughly diagnose illnesses than to treat them on an episodic basis.[81] Thus, by reimbursing physicians for the time spent caring for miners and their families, the Fund was able to promote managed care. For example, Fund administrators found that the slower pace of work at the Centerville Clinic relative to that at neighboring fee-for-service practices increased the thoroughness and accuracy of diagnoses. Centerville physicians spent more time with patients, saw fewer patients, used more ancillary personnel, and kept more extensive records. The clinic also had longer hours than competing fee-for-service providers. Yet, higher quality of care did not apparently result in higher costs. Centerville physicians' maximum salary of $38,200, paid out of the clinic retainer, was less than the average salary of $43,800 at local fee-for-service group practices. Moreover, Centerville had lower overhead and lower expenses per physician than its fee-for-service competitors.[82]

The retainer mechanism fulfilled another Fund objective by drawing qualified physicians to the coalfields. Many physicians were attracted by the prospect of being able to provide thorough and continuous routine care without fear of inadequate reimbursement. Fund administrators related that a physician at the Centerville Clinic who had previously practiced in Long Island, "stated his appreciation for the freedom afforded in the Centerville Clinic to work his patients up thoroughly, the lack of Fund interference in patient care, the absence of financial pressures and the ability to keep people ambulatory and out of the hospitals—something he could not accomplish under his previous Blue Cross-Blue Shield fee-for-service practice. Without a fee arrangement, he believes he can now give better care, with more time for individual patients."[83] Physicians like these appreciated retainer payments as another realization of the progressive approach sponsored by the Fund.[84]

The Fund made retainer arrangements with both individual practitioners and group practices. Hubert Marshall, the chief medical administrator at Morgantown remarked,

> Integrity, ability, and attitude were the major factors in determining the doctors to be approached in regards to accepting a retainer for their services to our beneficiaries. The amount paid these physicians was not a controlling factor in their selection. We had to be certain that the doctors

selected would give our beneficiaries adequate treatment without the feeling that they were being underpaid for their services or that the Fund was just a 'dole' and the majority of the patients could be given a few pills and sent home with the hope and expectation that they would contact another doctor if necessary.[85]

The AMOs negotiated retainer payments individually with each physician or group of physicians based on the amount of time they spent caring for Fund beneficiaries. Hence, retainer payments were often referred to as "fee-for-time" payments. In calculating physician fees, the AMOs applied the percentage of time the physician spent with Fund beneficiaries to the average physician income in the area.[86] The retainer also was calculated to cover the amount of the provider's overhead proportionate to the services it provided to Fund beneficiaries. Thus, the retainer was essentially a per capita payment based on the provider's total costs, resembling the payment scheme used by modern health maintenance organizations.

The Fund's payment method included a further deviation from the prevailing norm as, unlike that of traditional third-party payers, it was not based on fee schedules. Fund administrators felt that while schedules were intended to serve as fee ceilings, they more often rapidly became fee floors. Furthermore, the Fund felt that fee schedules did not allow for differences in training and ability among physicians, and in the severity of illness or injury among patients.[87] By contrast, the retainer payment system allowed for these differences while the reporting requirements and continual monitoring by the AMOs' staffs identified charges that were unreasonable.

In order to determine the appropriate retainer payment, the AMOs monitored physicians both before and after they were placed on retainer and mandated that retainer rates be subject to renegotiation at any time. The Fund required retainer physicians to keep a register of Fund patients and to submit monthly reports to the AMO. Provider requests for increases in retainers were awarded only when the AMO judged the increases to be justified based on its review of invoices and discussions with the provider. In instances where the charges were deemed to be unreasonable, the AMO encouraged providers to decrease their costs by, for instance, increasing their volume of patients or by increasing their use of ancillary personnel.[88] If such discussions did not result in lower charges, the AMO retained the right to drop the provider from its participating physician list.

Physicians involved in group practice typically formed a nonprofit entity to which the Fund paid the clinic's retainer. The physicians then determined the distribution of salaries among themselves.[89] For instance, physicians at the Centerville and Bellaire clinics determined individual physician shares of the group retainer based on the amount of time each physician spent with Fund patients, the physician's length of service with the group, and the physician's experience and training.[90] Retainer payments often comprised most of the funding for group practices in the coalfields. For example, the Russellton Clinic derived 57 percent of its income from Fund retainers, 15 percent from check-off payments (presumably from miners and their families among others), and 28 percent from fee-for-service patients.[91]

The retainer mechanism also resulted in considerable savings in administrative costs as compared to fee-for-service reimbursement. Paperwork was reduced since the Fund made only monthly or semimonthly payments to providers instead of processing each claim separately. Similarly, physicians' paperwork also decreased as they did not have to file separate claims for each service provided.[92] Furthermore, in return for the stability and predictability that the retainer payments provided, physicians often reduced the fees they charged the Fund by 10 to 15 percent.[93]

It should be noted that the retainer system did not fully guard against two problems inherent in medical care reimbursement: inaccurate disclosure of costs and cross-subsidization of non-beneficiaries. While all insurers face these problems, the Fund's monitoring mechanism made it easier to reduce the incidence of these events.

First, the Fund relied on providers to disclose services provided and their resulting costs accurately and honestly. The AMOs' practice of screening providers to determine whether they shared the Fund's philosophy increased the probability that physicians accepted for the retainer program would disclose costs accurately. Moreover, the Fund's continual review of provider records allowed the Fund to detect fraudulent behavior, to some degree. However, given that providers, and not the Fund directly, computed costs, the ability of providers to disclose costs inaccurately or dishonestly was not eradicated entirely. While there is little evidence of the extent of the Fund's concern about this issue, an internal Fund memo does note that non-profit clinics were more cooperative in disclosing financial data than were proprietary clinics.[94]

Second, concerns were raised within the Fund that the retainer payments often resulted in cross-subsidization of non-beneficiaries. For instance, where non-beneficiaries utilized physician services more intensively than beneficiaries, the clinic's resultant higher costs would be passed on to the Fund through the retainer payments. For example, 56 percent of the Russellton Clinic's patient base was comprised of miners and their families and this group contributed 72 percent of the clinic's income.[95] Certain Fund administrators felt that the costs to the Fund of cross-subsidization were offset by the benefits of continuing to encourage non-beneficiaries to visit providers that cared for Fund beneficiaries. Specifically, Newdorp argued that payments by non-beneficiaries helped cover the providers' overhead[96] and that the presence of non-beneficiaries expanded the diversity of the patient pool, allowing providers to expand their range of services.[97]

The Fund's reliance on the retainer method of payment varied by area and over time. The prevalence of the retainer system can be described by the percentage of the Fund's total physician payments in each area that went to retainer physicians. As shown in Table 9, retainer physicians received 15.6 percent of the Fund's total payments for all physician services in 1954, but by 1974, retainer physicians received 55.9 percent of total physician payments. The percentage of total physician payments devoted to retainers rose steadily throughout the period before the initiation of Medicare in July 1966. The heaviest use of retainer payments occurred in the Birmingham, Knoxville, Pittsburgh, Morgantown, and Charleston AMOs while retainer payments were less prevalent in the Louisville, Beckley, Denver, Johnstown, and St. Louis areas. Another measure of the extent of retainer payments is the number of physicians who were paid in this manner; in 1968 approximately 70 percent of the 8,000 physicians serving Fund beneficiaries were paid on retainer.[98]

The Fund had two principal goals in moving from fee-for-service reimbursement toward reimbursement by retainer. First, the Fund hoped that the stability of income provided by retainer payments would induce physicians to locate in the coalfields. Second, administrators expected retainer payments to increase efficiency of care. By not reimbursing providers for individual procedures, the retainer method removed the financial incentives of performing unnecessary surgery and hospitalization where other less costly treatments were available.[99] The results presented below provide evidence that retainer payments did, in fact, reduce hospitalization and provide care at a lower cost per beneficiary.

A sense of the use of retainer physicians can be obtained from the number of surgical cases, hospital calls, and office calls each provider reported.[100] Since only the absolute volume of calls was reported without information on the number of beneficiaries receiving care, the rates of this type of care cannot be determined precisely. However, it is safe to assume that the number of beneficiaries cared for by retainer physicians increased in this period due to the promotion of the program by Fund administrators.

Table 9 Retainer payments to physicians as a percentage of total payments to physicians in each AMO, 1954–1974

	1954	1958	1962	1966	1970	1974
Birmingham	61.5%	76.5%	85.5%	88.4%	87.4%	63.2%
Knoxville	23.2	43.6	64.3	76.2	89.0	74.1
Pittsburgh	22.0	60.3	73.6	75.4	60.0	54.6
Morgantown	15.0	57.5	75.5	73.0	62.4	58.0
Charleston	10.1	25.1	45.0	53.8	70.8	61.8
Louisville	0.0	0.2	26.4	42.2	81.7	59.7
Beckley	3.2	17.8	25.5	42.0	51.8	44.0
Denver	20.4	36.7	38.6	25.1	18.1	24.2
Johnstown	0.0	7.8	12.7	14.1	12.9	13.7
St. Louis	3.4	4.7	7.7	11.3	15.3	49.2
ALL AREAS	15.6%	36.8%	54.4%	56.5%	62.7%	55.9%

Source: UMWA Welfare and Retirement Fund, Office of Research and Statistics, "Summary of Retainers," various years, Fund Archives.

Administrators not only wanted to take advantage of the relative unit cost savings of retainer physicians cited previously, but also felt that retainer physicians were easier to monitor and control, given the reporting requirements of the program and the significance of Fund beneficiaries to these practices. In fact, the Fund's increasing reliance on retainer payments can be demonstrated by the percentage of total payments to physicians that went to those practicing on retainer. In the period before the inception of Medicare, the percentage of physician payments received by retainer physicians increased steadily from 15.6 percent in 1954, to 57.3 percent in 1965.[101]

Figure 2 displays the number of hospital and office calls provided by all retainer physicians.[102] After an initial increase in both office and hospital calls, presumably due to the initial recruitment of physicians to the program, the number of calls leveled off from the mid-1950s to the early 1960s.[103] Beginning in 1960, the number of office calls increased much more rapidly than that of hospital calls. Without information on the rate of calls per beneficiary, it is difficult to explain these trends fully. However, it is quite likely that the rise in office calls that occurred without a concomitant rise in hospital calls was due to either a shift in the provision of care to treatment in the physicians' office at earlier stages of illness or a relatively greater dependence on ambulatory provision of surgery.[104] This outcome is apparent upon closer examination of retainer payments in northern Appalachia. Retainer payments were used most extensively in this region, taking advantage of the availability of well-established, reliable group prac-

Figure 2   Number of hospital and office calls provided by all Fund retainer physicians, 1953–1974

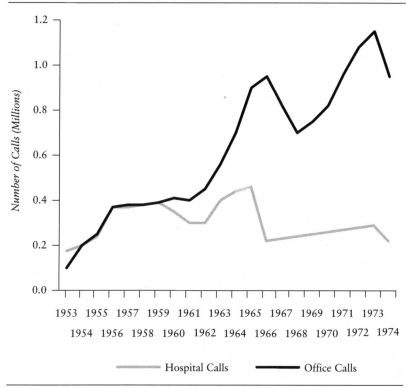

Source: Office of Research and Statistics, "Summary of Retainers," various years, Fund Archives.

tices.[105] Group practices are better positioned than solo practitioners to substitute office care for hospital care.

The benefits of the retainer program were quickly realized. In 1954 the Fund studied sixteen specialists in the Pittsburgh AMO, eight who were paid on retainer and eight who were reimbursed on a fee-for-service basis.[106] First, the study found that fee-for-service physicians tended to make more calls, possibly because of their financial incentive to provide more service.[107] Second, fee-for-service physicians charged somewhat more per call, in part because fee-for-service physicians had a greater tendency to treat their patients in hospitals instead of in their offices. This was particularly true in internal medicine where the cost per case was 63 percent higher under fee-for-service arrangements. Third, the study showed that fee-for-service physicians were more likely to perform surgery. For example, in the case of gynecological patients, retainer physicians reported surgery in 28 percent of their cases while fee-for-service physicians reported surgery in 68 percent of their cases. Eager to benefit further from the use of retainer payments, the Pittsburgh area increased its use of retainer physicians so that by 1955 they received 19 percent of all payments to physicians, and by 1956 they received 52 percent of all physician payments.[108]

Ample data exist to evaluate the success of this program beyond the early 1950s. Since the AMOs reimbursed retainer physicians based on the amount of service they provided, a wealth of information on the costs of the program is available. Specifically, the AMOs collected extensive data on the absolute volume of care provided by retainer physicians and the magnitude of retainer payments in relation to fee-for-service payments. However, evidence on utilization is somewhat incomplete as no information exists on the number of beneficiaries receiving care from retainer physicians. As a result, the rates of usage for various types of care provided by retainer physicians cannot be determined precisely.

The AMOs used the information they collected on the total fees charged by retainer physicians to construct two indicators of the cost of retainer charges relative to fee-for-service charges. The first measure (used from 1953 to 1966) employed a proxy, called the "evaluation," to represent a hypothetical fee-for-service charge for a level of service comparable to that provided by the retainer physician. The evaluation was obtained by multiplying the number of office and hospital calls by a standard fee for each. The standard fees were adjusted periodically to account for inflation.[109] The fee paid was then divided by the evaluation, providing a ratio of the actual retainer payment to the hypothetical fee-for-service payment. For example, in 1958 the ratio of the retainer fee to the evaluation was 0.81. Hence, by using retainer payments the Fund paid only 81 percent of what it would have paid had the retainer physicians had been reimbursed on a fee-for-service basis. From 1953 until 1966, the overall Fund ratio of retainer payments to hypothetical fee-for-service payments ranged from 0.81 to 1.11, averaging 0.94 with a standard deviation of 0.08 (see Figure 3).[110] Thus by this measure the Fund realized, on average, a 6 percent savings through the use of retainer payments.

From 1967 to 1974, the Fund reported a different measure to compare retainer payments to fee-for-service reimbursement.[111] Here, the actual fee paid was divided by the number of hospital and office calls (with hospital calls weighted higher) to obtain a measure of the "cost per unit of service." This measure provided a set of fees that allowed the Fund to make com-

Figure 3 Ratio of total Fund retainer fees to evaluations, 1953–1966

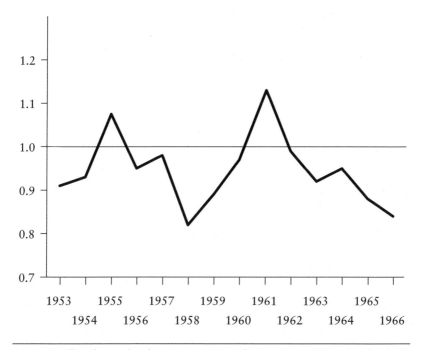

Source: Office of Research and Statistics, "Summary of Retainers," various years, Fund Archives.

parisons within the pool of retainer providers. The advantage of this measure is that it avoids the arbitrariness of employing one "standard" fee to construct an evaluation. While the Fund only reported this measure after 1966, data exist to calculate the cost per unit for the period from 1953 to 1966, as shown in Figure 4. The similarities between Figures 3 and 4 suggest that the two measures of the relative costs of the two payment mechanisms provide comparable results.

These two measures show that the Fund was successful in containing costs through the use of retainer payments at least in the period before the inception of Medicare in 1966. From 1953 to 1966, the ratios of fees paid to evaluation remained below one for all but two years (1955 and 1961), suggesting that throughout this period the Fund saved money by using retainer payments. During this same period, the cost per unit of service increased only moderately and actually exhibited a decline in the 1960s. It is more difficult to evaluate the Fund's success in containing physician costs

Figure 4 Average cost per unit of service provided by all Fund retainer
physicians, 1953–1974

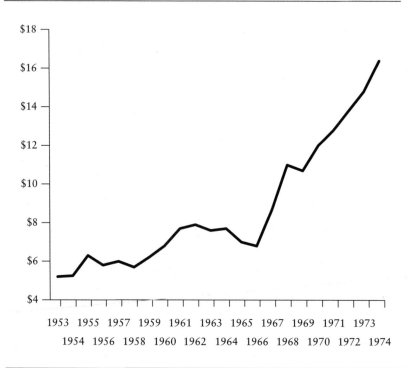

Note: cost per unit = $\dfrac{\text{Retainer Fee}}{1.5 \times (\text{Hospital Calls}) + (\text{Office Calls})}$

Source: Office of Research and Statistics, "Summary of Retainers," various years, Fund Archives.

in the period after the inception of Medicare in 1966. The cost per unit
escalated rapidly after 1966, but in the absence of evidence on the level of
prevailing fees elsewhere, it is not possible to determine how this increase
compared to the general rise in physician fees.

The Fund reaped significant savings in the cost of physician care through
the use of retainer payments. The retainer program was most successful in
AMOs where physicians sympathetic to the Fund's attention to costs were
available to care for a significant volume of Fund beneficiaries. Besides rendering significant cost savings, the retainer payments also provided stable
income to providers operating in communities where funds for health care
were otherwise scarce. The guaranteed income provided by retainer payments was a crucial component in the continued operation and development

of group practices as well as in the retention of physicians recruited to work in the coalfields. In fact, anecdotal evidence suggests that the stability of income afforded by retainer payments encouraged many providers to offer the Fund discounts for their services, thus contributing further cost savings.

Finally, without precise participation statistics, it is difficult to determine the extent of the contribution of retainer payments to reductions in the hospitalization rates of beneficiaries. It is quite possible that the contribution was significant in areas most dependent on retainer physicians. Most notably, retainer payments were particularly prevalent in northern and southern Appalachia AMOs which also experienced low relative discharge rates. Similarly, within central Appalachia, Charleston used retainer payments to a greater extent than any other area in the region and also had the lowest discharge rate in the region.

In areas where they were used extensively, the use of retainer payments provided the Fund with cost savings that were greater and endured longer than those provided by the cut in the participating physicians list. Moreover, the savings occurred without a reduction in the quality of care. In fact, quality of care most likely increased with the use of retainer payments as physicians were less likely to engage in unnecessary surgery and hospitalization. Furthermore, since they were reimbursed for the time they spent with beneficiaries, physicians were not tempted to sacrifice time diagnosing and treating individual beneficiaries in order to increase their volume of patients. Finally, the benefits of the retainer program accrued despite the usual obstacles present in caring for a group of beneficiaries with considerable medical needs. As such, the retainer program suggests a model for physician payment that has applications beyond this setting.

In less than a decade, the administrators of the Welfare and Retirement Fund had developed a comprehensive health care plan that deviated radically from mainstream medical care. Guided by their resolute belief that managed care would raise standards of care while holding down costs, Fund administrators sought to create incentives that would prompt providers to supply appropriate treatment at reasonable prices. Faced with physician shortages, the administrators recruited qualified physicians to the coalfields. Unwilling to tolerate scarce, substandard hospital facilities, the Fund helped develop group practices to provide outpatient care and, as will be discussed in chapter 5, built its own state-of-the-art hospitals. Where most health care experts saw desolation, Fund administrators saw the opportunity to create a modern health care system.

There can be little doubt that the Fund was successful in improving the access to and the quality of care received by coal miners and their families.

The AMOs' careful monitoring and review of providers eradicated company doctors who provided unacceptable care or charged unreasonable fees. By developing the health care infrastructure in the coalfields, the Fund eliminated the intolerable system of care documented in the Boone Report.

The Fund's record as far as increasing the cost-effectiveness of care is concerned is more difficult to evaluate precisely. At least two of the Fund's initiatives produced discernible cost savings. The cut in the participating physicians list in 1957 resulted in immediate, albeit temporary, decreases in utilization and costs. The retainer payment system produced cost savings throughout its period of use. However, while the Fund may have registered some savings through these programs, its beneficiaries continued to use hospitals at higher rates than did non-beneficiaries living in the same regions. This result is consistent with the bias toward hospital care inherent in the Fund's coverage. In the absence of coverage for routine primary care and with the presence of high quality of care available through Fund-sponsored specialists and hospitals, high hospital admission rates are not surprising.

Yet the high hospitalization rates may also have resulted from characteristics of the beneficiaries and of the mining regions. First, Fund beneficiaries had relatively greater health needs that, not surprisingly, suggest that they would also use hospitals more intensively. Second, the scarcity of alternatives to hospital care in particularly underdeveloped parts of the coalfields also contributed to high rates of hospitalization. Moreover, beneficiaries' high relative usage may have been a consequence, to some degree, of underutilization by non-beneficiaries. These considerations imply, therefore, that beneficiaries' *high* hospitalization rates should not be viewed solely as *excessive* utilization rates.

Perhaps the greatest strength of the Fund's program was its administrators' ability to eschew ad hoc attempts to influence physician behavior and instead fashion initiatives that complemented each other and worked together as part of an overall package. As a physician who had participated in the Fund's program wrote to Lorin Kerr, "my move from Harlan to Louisville has been like going from an oasis into the middle of the desert. Louisville has no groups, no one attempting to provide comprehensive medical care, and only the traditional episodic illness-fee for service situation. Since most people do not have health insurance, this results in marked overutilization of existing hospital beds. I am sure the pattern is well-known to you."[112] The suggestion that Harlan, located in the heart of Appalachia, provided a more progressive medical care environment than the urban metropolis of Louisville attests to the impact of the Fund's efforts in reforming the provision of physician care.

CHAPTER FIVE

Hospital Care: The Miners Memorial Hospital Association

*I*n many ways, the culmination of the Fund's managed care initiatives as a whole was the establishment of its own chain of hospitals in the heart of Appalachia. As early as 1951, top Fund administrators began discussing the prospect of constructing and operating a chain of hospitals in order to extend further the Fund's ability to coordinate a comprehensive array of services. Specifically, Fund administrators hoped that by operating their own set of hospitals, they could achieve two objectives: to increase the supply of hospital care that met the Fund's quality standards and to attract qualified physicians to work in underserved areas.[1]

The ten hospitals that the Fund opened in late 1955 and early 1956 unequivocally succeeded in achieving the two objectives. The Miners Memorial Hospitals brought an unprecedented level of hospital care to Appalachia and attracted prominent physicians eager to participate in this bold venture. The hospitals were instrumental in raising the standards of hospital care in the coalfields by introducing state-of-the-art equipment, outpatient care, and specialty services. In addition, the Fund sponsored innovations in the administration and remuneration of the physician staffs at the hospitals.

Despite the national attention they received, the Miners Hospitals were the first of the Fund's managed care initiatives to be abandoned. In large part, the Fund's lack of success in controlling the cost of hospitalization would eventually doom the project. What Fund administrators failed to appreciate fully was the high cost of providing such care, especially in an era when the beneficiary population was declining. In addition, Fund trustees proved to be unwilling to continue supporting the hospitals when they failed to be filled with Fund beneficiaries. This chapter will describe the evolution of the hospital chain and will evaluate its success in achieving its objectives. This discussion provides the background necessary to evaluate the trustees' decision to sell the chain described in chapter 6.

The Fund constructed its own hospitals to address the undersupply of hospitals in the coalfields that met their quality standards. In some areas with particularly high concentrations of mining families, there were absolutely no local hospitals. In areas where local hospitals did exist, they were often unacceptable to Fund administrators. In Appalachia in particular, the Fund was forced to rely heavily on private hospitals known to charge excessive fees for low quality service.[2] Conditions apparently had not changed much since the Boone Report as Fund administrators found that many miners and their families continued to have access to only substandard hospital facilities and unsanitary hospital conditions. In fact—a possibility that apparently went unnoticed by Fund administrators—the Fund's reimbursement policy itself may have increased the level of substandard care. Physicians lacking either the qualifications or the resources to operate a hospital may have entered the market in order to take advantage of Fund reimbursement for hospital and specialist care. For example, physicians were reported to have converted mansions into "hospitals," possibly solely to receive Fund compensation.[3]

Moreover, the Fund found that non-staff physicians often could not obtain admitting privileges at private hospitals.[4] Often, it was precisely those physicians that the Fund felt could best provide quality care—physicians who endorsed the Fund's policies—that were prevented from treating patients in these hospitals. In effect, then, the inferior conditions in many hospitals could not be mitigated by having the patients cared for by an attending physician the Fund found trustworthy. In fact, in some areas the Fund's relationship with the medical societies that dictated the policies of these hospitals grew so hostile that the it felt that the only way to ensure that beneficiaries received acceptable hospital care was to provide care in its own hospitals.[5]

As early as 1951, the Fund began a detailed examination of the state of hospital care in the coalfields in order to determine which areas suffered the greatest deficit of quality hospital care. For example, when Fund administrators surveyed the Beckley area in central Appalachia they found that there was not only a general shortage of hospital beds, but also a shortage of acceptable beds. Of the five hospitals in the area, the Fund determined that only two, and to a limited extent a third, provided acceptable services. This left a shortage of 390 acceptable beds, or 278 beds if unacceptable beds were included. In addition, the administrators noted that the existing hospitals employed closed staff arrangements which deterred physicians from locating in the Beckley area and, thus, hampered the development of high quality medical care there. This was especially problematic given the area's urgent need for specialists.[6]

Based on the surveys of hospital care in the coalfields and discussions between administrators, the Fund eventually settled on 10 strategically located sites—home to one-third of the UMWA membership[7]—for the construction of its hospitals: the Kentucky towns of Harlan, Hazard, Middlesboro, Pikeville, McDowell, and Whitesburg; the West Virginia towns of Beckley, Man, and Williamson; and the Virginia town of Wise (see Map 3). The Fund spent $30 million of its own funds to construct the hospitals.[8] Administrators felt that it was crucial to invest in plant and equipment of a high caliber in order to be able to provide the level of care needed to serve beneficiaries adequately and to attract physicians to Appalachia. Heeding a suggestion of the Boone Report, the Fund created a nonprofit corporation, the Miners Memorial Hospital Association (MMHA), to own and operate the chain of hospitals. Continuing its practice of enlisting the services of prominent health experts, the Fund hired Dr. Fred Mott, the former deputy minister of health in Saskatchewan and an expert in rural health systems, to head the MMHA.[9] He was succeeded by Dr. John Newdorp in 1957.

The hospitals dramatically increased the supply of hospital beds by providing 1,085 new beds to the region.[10] For instance, the Beckley Memorial Hospital's 207 beds accounted for 21.2 percent of Fund beneficiary admissions in the Beckley area and 29.9 percent of the beneficiaries' short-term hospital days in 1958 as shown in Table 10. By 1964, Beckley Memorial would provide 33.0 percent of the area's beneficiary admissions and 39.4 percent of its beneficiaries' hospital days.[11] It should be noted that the MMHA hospitals were open to patients not covered by the Fund and, on average, roughly one-fourth of the chain's beds were occupied by non-beneficiaries.

Table 11 displays the absolute number of admission and the absolute number of outpatient visits to MMHA hospitals from their first full year of operation in 1956 to their sale in 1963 and 1964. After an initial increase in admissions following the opening of the hospitals, total admissions to most hospitals leveled off or fell in the ensuing years. However, while admissions did not grow significantly, the percentage of Fund beneficiaries cared for in the Memorial Hospitals in the four areas where they were located did increase. By 1962, as shown in Table 12, the MMHA cared for from roughly a third to two-thirds of all hospital services provided to beneficiaries in central Appalachia. The Knoxville AMO managed to place the greatest proportion of hospital patients in Memorial Hospitals, roughly doubling their share of discharges and days from 1957 to 1962 to the point

Map 3 Location of MMHA hospitals and Fund AMOs

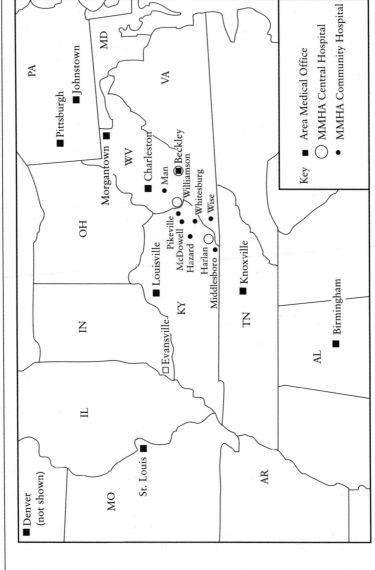

Table 10 Service provided to Fund beneficiaries by Beckley Memorial
Hospital as compared to service provided by all short-term
hospitals in the Beckley AMO, 1958–1966

	1958	*1960*	*1962*	*1964ᵃ*	*1966ᵃ*
Hospital Admissions to Beckley Memorial	4,541	4,685	4,719	5,009	4,095
Hospital Admissions to Beckley Memorial as a % of the Area's Total Admissions	21.2%	23.9%	30.8%	33.0%	29.6%
Hospital Days of Care at Beckley Memorial	52,418	48,733	50,760	47,630	33,662
Hospital Days of Care at Beckley Memorial as a % of the Area's Total Days of Care	29.9%	30.4%	40.6%	39.4%	33.8%

ᵃFigures are for Memorial Hospitals after their sale to ARHI.

Source: UMWA Welfare and Retirement Fund Collection, Office of Research and Statistics, "Hospital Service to Fund Beneficiaries," various years, Fund Archives.

where more than half of the hospital service in the area was provided by Memorial Hospitals.

The MMHA hospitals provided critical outpatient services in areas where facilities for ambulatory care and diagnostic services were typically as scarce as hospital facilities. Table 11 shows that the majority of MMHA hospitals managed to increase their provision of outpatient services during their time of operation. Fund administrators were particularly eager to promote outpatient services as a substitute for more costly hospital care. Given that the hospitals were constructed in a region with an underdeveloped medical infrastructure, the outpatient clinics provided services that elsewhere might have been supplied by group practices.

The Fund aimed to coordinate hospital care both within the chain and within the health care plan as a whole. First, the hospitals acted as an integrated unit, directed by a single administration that set uniform policies. Within the chain, the three hospitals at Beckley, Williamson, and Harlan acted as central hospitals that provided the widest possible range of service. The remaining seven hospitals served as satellite hospitals that provided standard care and referred more complicated cases to the central hospitals (see Map 4).[12]

Table 11 Admissions, average lengths–of–stay, and outpatient visits, MMHA hospitals, 1956–1963

	All MMHA	Beckley	Harlan	Williamson	Whitesburg	Man	Hazard	Middlesboro	McDowell	Wise	Pikeville
Admissions											
1956	26,988	4,504	4,098	2,905	2,321	2,588	2,715	1,969	2,149	1,887	1,852
1957	26,694	5,346	4,283	3,820	2,257	2,556	2,875	2,443	2,079	1,946	2,089
1958	31,299	5,649	4,678	3,732	2,192	2,530	3,258	2,949	1,945	2,072	2,294
1959	30,368	5,851	4,646	3,463	1,940	2,635	2,711	2,763	1,865	2,333	2,161
1960	29,006	6,029	4,239	3,635	1,770	2,707	2,325	2,501	1,707	2,078	2,015
1961	31,376	6,097	4,493	4,046	2,519	2,991	2,017	2,671	2,000	2,366	2,176
1962	27,965	5,850	4,286	3,435	1,905	2,805	1,823	2,602	1,484	2,097	1,678
1963	34,034	6,902	5,586	3,908	2,418	3,121	2,832	3,240	1,893	2,353	1,781
Length-of–Stay (days)											
1956	9.1	12.7	10.5	10.7	8.5	7.4	6.2	8.5	6.5	7.7	6.8
1957	9.2	11.3	11.2	10.6	9.4	8.3	6.4	8.0	7.4	8.1	6.4
1958	9.1	10.8	12.0	10.6	9.8	7.8	5.7	7.7	7.1	7.9	6.2
1959	9.1	10.4	11.7	10.8	8.6	8.1	6.4	8.2	7.2	7.8	6.6
1960	9.0	9.8	12.8	10.5	7.0	7.7	6.0	8.3	7.1	8.2	6.4
1961	9.7	10.0	12.7	11.5	9.0	7.5	10.4	9.0	8.2	8.3	6.3
1962	10.0	10.4	12.7	11.6	12.0	7.7	10.9	7.8	7.1	8.1	7.2
1963	8.2	9.2	9.3	10.1	7.1	7.3	7.1	6.5	6.6	8.1	6.2

Table 11 Continued

	All MMHA	Beckley	Harlan	Williamson	Whitesburg	Man	Hazard	Middlesboro	McDowell	Wise	Pikeville
Outpatient Visits											
1956	202,313	43,673	25,588	18,894	16,479	23,539	17,030	23,205	18,658	14,859	3,388
1957	271,139	58,968	28,723	34,418	22,578	30,515	20,092	25,607	25,036	17,197	8,005
1958	350,871	74,141	39,943	43,391	27,239	38,447	28,393	29,501	27,565	17,128	25,123
1959	393,168	74,706	45,875	51,677	27,941	43,423	28,546	34,344	29,092	24,151	33,413
1960	389,971	73,336	40,014	48,538	28,240	48,068	25,355	30,712	27,790	26,558	35,360
1961	412,798	74,692	51,070	52,295	24,977	53,099	24,597	33,574	32,342	29,160	36,992
1962	368,836	70,875	48,920	52,171	21,407	45,621	18,730	29,565	27,236	27,342	29,969
1963	346,965	69,381	46,287	55,780	12,731	47,396	2,267	23,180	32,219	30,836	26,888

Note: Years represent fiscal years from October 1 of the year listed to September 31 of the following year.

Source: UMWA Office of Research and Statistics, "MMHA—Summary Statistics," various years, Fund Archives.

Table 12   Percentage of short-term hospital cases and hospital days in each
AMO cared for in MMHA hospitals, 1957–1963

| | Hospital cases | | | | | | |
	1957	*1958*	*1959*	*1960*	*1961*	*1962*	*1963*
Beckley	15.9%	21.1%	20.2%	23.8%	29.2%	26.8%	
Charleston	22.0	27.9	29.5	31.5	38.5	43.7	
Knoxville	29.1	33.3	37.1	39.4	46.8	54.8	
Louisville	28.7	36.1	36.6	35.8	37.9	39.0	
ALL AREAS	14.5%	17.6%	18.5%	18.8%	21.5%	23.0%	22.3%

| | Hospital days | | | | | | |
	1957	*1958*	*1959*	*1960*	*1961*	*1962*	*1963*
Beckley	24.7%	29.5%	29.6%	31.0%	38.9%	35.6%	
Charleston	25.3	36.5	35.7	37.0	42.1	48.7	
Knoxville	34.6	43.3	48.4	51.6	62.2	67.6	
Louisville	29.2	36.2	36.4	34.8	34.3	40.2	
ALL AREAS	15.5%	19.7%	20.3%	20.4%	22.6%	27.1%	27.8%

Source: UMWA Office of Research and Statistics, "Statistical Report," various years, Fund
Archives.

Second, in addition to coordinating services within the hospital chain,
the Fund attempted to coordinate the care provided by the MMHA with
the its other objectives. This effort was most explicit in determining the
funding for the hospitals. The Fund's national office negotiated the hospitals' annual budgets through discussions with the MMHA.[13] A report on
one of the first such sets of budget negotiations stated, "The [Budget]
Committee meetings emphasized the necessity of teamwork to bring unit
costs down so that the hospitals will provide more services to more beneficiaries. The importance of integration of the services of provided by the
MMHA with the medical care administration of the Fund was emphasized
repeatedly."[14]

In addition to controlling costs in MMHA hospitals, the Fund was also
concerned with reducing its reliance on other non-MMHA hospitals where
its own hospitals were available. Integrating the MMHA into its operations
allowed the Fund to promote efforts to decrease the use of less favorable
hospitals. Based on their frequent reviews of the utilization rates of the
Memorial Hospitals, in the fall of 1958 the medical directors of the AMOs
that included Memorial Hospitals in their jurisdiction (Beckley, Louisville,
Knoxville, and Charleston) informed Draper of the losses the Fund was sus-

Map 4 Location of Central and Community MMHA hospitals

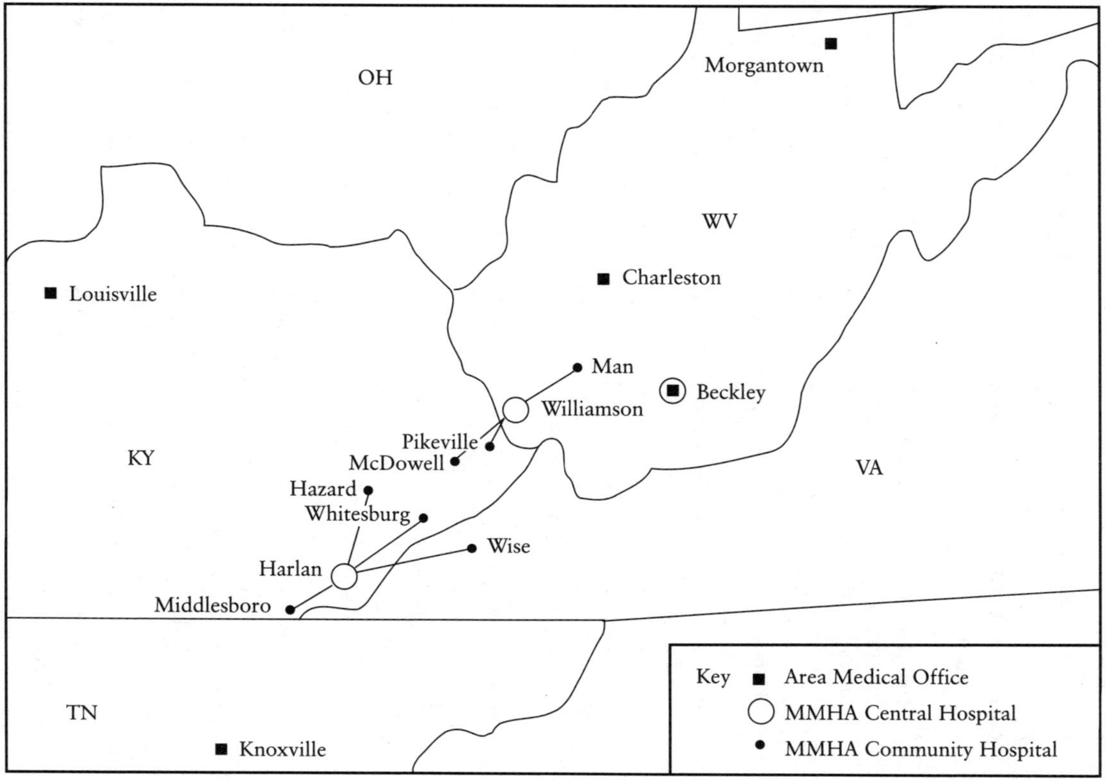

Key
- ■ Area Medical Office
- ◎ MMHA Central Hospital
- • MMHA Community Hospital

OH

KY

WV

VA

TN

Louisville ■

Morgantown ■

Charleston ■

Man •

Williamson ◎

Beckley ◎

Pikeville •

McDowell •

Hazard •

Whitesburg •

Wise •

Harlan ◎

Middlesboro •

Knoxville ■

taining by failing to fully use the hospitals for care of Fund beneficiaries. In addition, the administrators identified ten specific competing hospitals in their areas to which they were especially interested in curtailing or eliminating services.[15]

The coordination of the MMHA with the Fund extended beyond the provision of hospital care to include the development of a comprehensive range of care in underserved areas. For example, in 1958 Draper recommended to Newdorp:

> That Dr. Winebrenner [the administrator of the Knoxville AMO] be authorized to encourage the establishment of one or more new group clinics in the Dante-Clintwood-Grundy area where a number of new mines have been opened. General practitioners who could be obtained to join such groups, with specialist consultants from the Memorial Hospitals, would divert many patients to the Wise Memorial Hospital and our cooperating hospital at Norton. They are now being referred by the doctors in these areas to hospitals in Bristol and Abingdon. These are the doctors who provide them with home and office care and upon whom they are dependent; also, the Bristol and Abingdon hospitals are more accessible than the hospital at Wise. Dr. Winebrenner is confident that he could get such clinics established at no cost to the Fund if he were sure we were willing that he do so.[16]

The Fund, therefore, was able to capitalize on the Memorial Hospitals' services to enhance the level of physician care in the surrounding areas. This arrangement also served the Fund's aim of reducing its reliance on competing hospitals.

What is clear from these examples is that the MMHA was not intended to act as an independent provider of hospital services to the Fund. While encouraged to provide the highest possible level of service, the Memorial Hospitals were not given unfettered control over their operations. Rather, as part of a larger system of care, each hospital was expected to subordinate its own individual interests to the advancement of the interests of the system as a whole.

The Memorial Hospitals' high level of care was due in part to the range of care they provided. Unique among Appalachian hospitals, the MMHA hospitals sponsored outpatient clinics, specialty services, and ongoing research and education efforts. The Fund's concern for cost control resulted in its pioneering campaign for the provision of outpatient and ambulatory care wherever appropriate. Besides providing the type of services typically associated with outpatient clinics—minor surgery, therapy, and testing—

these clinics also provided a considerable degree of routine physician care. Regions that lacked adequate hospital care (like those where the Miners Hospitals were erected) were also likely to have inadequate physician care. This was of concern to the Fund since patients were likely to visit a hospital for routine care if adequate physician care was unavailable. The provision of routine care in hospitals was one of the outcomes that the Fund hoped to avoid by operating its own hospitals. Hence, even though the Fund did not cover routine physician care, it created outpatient clinics to provide this care in response to the potential for beneficiaries to seek hospital care in their absence.[17]

The hospital-based clinics followed the Fund's practice of charging for routine care. This policy proved to be problematic due to the price sensitivity of the beneficiaries. First, local physicians often did not charge for routine care. Instead, the cost of this care was recouped, in many cases, by recommending hospitalization that was later reimbursed by the Fund. As beneficiaries took advantage of this "free" care, they were more likely to later undergo expensive and unnecessary courses of treatment at the expense of the Fund. Hence by charging fees, the outpatient clinics weakened their potential for reducing hospitalization.

Second, the price sensitivity of beneficiaries was such that even a seemingly minor increase in fees from, say, $1 to $2 per visit would deter patients from seeking care, thus increasing their chances of needing more costly treatment later.[18] This problem is clearly demonstrated by the experience of the outpatient clinic at the Pikeville Memorial Hospital. Pikeville Memorial found that the large volume of walk-ins after hours produced by its Saturday clinic was severely taxing its staff. To reduce the number of after-hours walk-ins, Pikeville administrators increased the charge for non-emergency visits after clinic hours to $5 and reduced the charge for visits during regular hours from $3 to $2. This price differential reduced the after-hours patient volume by 40 percent. The administrators justified their actions by maintaining that the increase in charges after hours was not a intended to be a "penalty," but rather a method to encourage patients to use services wisely so as not to overburden staff.[19]

The fact that patient volume at the clinic had decreased substantially after the modest price increase was, however, not what makes this example particularly interesting. In fact, the Pikeville administrators had based their actions on similar adjustments made at the McDowell Memorial Hospital which had produced a comparable set of results. What makes this example noteworthy is the subsequent evaluation of the policy change by top Fund administrators. The Pikeville administrators informed Draper, in a rather self-congratulatory fashion, of their actions and their success in reducing after-hours visits. After discussing the matter with local union officials, Draper replied to the clinic that he was unconvinced that the $5 charge was desirable for a number of reasons. Draper argued that the increase in the daytime volume produced by the differential forced those people who came during the day to endure long waits. Moreover, he noted that many patients had good reasons for not visiting the clinic during regular hours or without an appointment. For instance, given their lack of medical knowledge, patients would believe they were in need of emergency care even though the clinic's staff could later conclude otherwise. In light of these concerns, then, Draper asked the clinic to discontinue the price differential.[20]

In general, administrators at the Fund's national office were convinced that educating clinic users was superior to erecting financial barriers to modify their behavior. John Newdorp, the MMHA's director, admonished physicians at the Whitesburg Clinic for treating walk-ins as "second class citizens" as revealed in interviews with patients. He noted that these patients were most likely accustomed to country doctors who practiced "almost anywhere they could set down their little black bag." Newdorp suggested that the clinic educate their patients so that its service could improve with their help, instead of despite their behavior.[21] Despite the difficulties of handling patients unfamiliar with their operations, the outpatient clinics appear to have provided a level of care commensurate with Fund standards. Physicians at the Beckley Memorial Hospital reported that they all worked in the outpatient clinic where they were "as interested in their outpatients as they are in those occupying beds."[22]

The quality of routine care provided in their outpatient clinics was complemented by the hospitals' provision of specialty services. For example, the Harlan Memorial Hospital provided plastic surgery service of a caliber that was practically unavailable elsewhere in Appalachia. The supply of such services not only increased the range of care available to beneficiaries, but also addressed the MMHA's need to increase utilization. As Newdorp explained,

> We find that patients are willing to travel great distances to avail themselves of something of a special nature which is not available locally. On the other hand, our attempts to simply transfer long-term patients on the basis that we have more space at one hospital than another, have not been successful since we have nothing additional to offer such patients as an incentive to go to a point far distant from their homes and friends.[23]

The ability of the Memorial Hospitals—particularly the three central hospitals—to attract patients in need of specialty services had repercussions for their admission rates and average lengths-of-stay. By treating the most critically ill and injured beneficiaries in a relatively more intensive way than competing hospitals, the Memorial Hospitals came to more closely resemble teaching hospitals with their high rates of admissions and longer stays. The resultant high costs of such care had consequences for the contribution of the MMHA hospitals to the Fund's drive for cost-effective care (see below).

Finally, the range of care offered by the Memorial Hospitals was enhanced continually by their ongoing research and education efforts. The Fund provided monies for research projects, including the study of black lung disease, undertaken at the hospitals. Outside grants provided additional funds for these efforts. The presence of medical residents at the hospitals created links to new treatment procedures developed at medical schools. The MMHA also organized a number of schools at the hospitals in order to train sorely needed medical personnel; a school to train nurses was established at the Williamson Memorial Hospital and a facility to train technicians was founded at the Beckley Memorial Hospital.[24]

The Fund organized and reimbursed physicians at the Memorial Hospitals in roughly the same unorthodox manner as it did the physicians in the group practices it sponsored. Looking first to the local stock of physicians, the Fund hired those physicians who were "qualified, competent, and willing to serve."[25] Given the large number of physicians that the hospitals required, the Fund also was obliged to recruit outside physicians to work in the MMHA hospitals. The effort to recruit physicians was begun in 1954 (a full two years before the hospitals opened) by the MMHA's clinical director, Dr. Aims McGuiness, a noted Philadelphia physician who had just resigned as the dean of University of Pennsylvania Graduate School of Medicine. McGuiness enlisted a sizable number of physicians with impressive credentials to join the Memorial Hospitals. The fact that more than half of the physicians were board-certified was significant given that they were assigned to areas that previously had only a handful of physicians with such qualifications.[26]

MMHA physicians were paid in a manner similar to group practice physicians. The physicians were not paid directly by the Fund but, instead, formed a Medical Associates organization which received payments from the Fund in the same manner as other retainer providers: in the form of a per capita assessment based on discussions concerning costs. The Medical

Associates organization—which operated system-wide and not by hospital— then distributed salaries to the physicians based on their experience, training, and length of service. Full-time staff salaries ranged from $12,000 per year for general practitioners to a maximum of $30,000 for specialists.[27] In some instances, special allowances were made to overcome particularly severe isolation and other disadvantages at certain hospitals. For example, to compensate physicians practicing at the McDowell Memorial Hospital, the Fund approved a $1,000 annual bonus with an additional $1,000 bonus per dependent child (not to exceed $3,000) and also purchased a house to be rented to the chief of clinical services.[28]

The MMHA also allowed its staff physicians to attend to non-beneficiaries receiving care in the hospitals, as long as these services did not interfere with the services provided to beneficiaries.[29] Payments received for the care of non-beneficiaries were deposited in the "special doctors' fund" at each hospital and were disbursed by hospital's medical staff.[30] This policy allowed physicians to care for non-beneficiaries but removed the incentives for personal gain that may have encouraged physicians to give priority to these patients. Finally, given the lack of specialists in the areas where the Memorial Hospitals were located, the MMHA allowed specialists on its staff to serve as consultants for beneficiaries receiving care at non-MMHA hospitals.[31]

As a whole, the ten hospitals employed 165 full-time, salaried staff physicians with slightly more than half acting as active staff members and the remaining physicians acting as consultative staff members. In addition, the MMHA granted courtesy privileges to 69 outside physicians. Beckley Memorial Hospital, the most heavily utilized MMHA hospital, employed 30 full-time salaried physicians—23 of whom were local physicians—on its active medical staff, granted an additional 15 local physicians courtesy privileges, retained seven outside consulting physicians to provide services as needed, and employed 13 residents.[32]

The volume of care provided by the Memorial Hospitals helped meet a critical need for quality hospital care in the coalfields. The Memorial Hospitals not only provided crucially needed beds, but also raised the standards for hospital care in central Appalachia. The hospitals were modern facilities with state-of-the-art equipment and staffs imported from preeminent medical centers in the United States. This premium level of care came, however, at a considerable price. Just a few years after the hospitals opened their doors, the cost of care at the Memorial Hospitals had reached unsustainable levels. Concurrently, fewer and fewer beneficiaries received care at the hospitals as Fund eligibility was tightened and employment levels in union mines fell (see chapter 6). Initially, attention to costs remained out of the spotlight as the trustees set their sights on building a group of facilities that would physically embody the achievements of the Fund, and the administrators absorbed themselves in raising the level of hospital care in the coalfields. Unlike other Fund initiatives, the design of the MMHA did not explicitly incorporate cost-control mechanisms. The Fund expected, at a minimum, to keep costs in the Memorial Hospitals in line with hospital costs elsewhere. However, there is no indication that administrators expected the chain to deliver cost-savings from, say, improving the integration and coordination of medical care.[33]

The fact that the Fund did not give cost control the same emphasis as the attainment of the highest possible quality of care does not mean that administrators ignored the level of costs in the hospitals. For instance, concerns over costs at the Memorial Hospitals were repeatedly expressed in the MMHA's annual budget reports. However, it appears that the speed with which costs reached crisis levels caught administrators by surprise. By 1960, cost over-runs were so high that administrators quickly became consumed with controlling costs as their top priority.

Complete information on costs at the Memorial Hospitals is not available but evidence of the magnitude of the problem administrators faced does exist. As early as 1957, administrators surveying conditions at the Memorial Hospitals expressed concern that average costs per day at the hospitals ranged between $30 and $80 as compared to the average community hospital charge of $20.[34] As a consequence of these relatively high charges, administrators found that the Memorial Hospitals created a drain on Fund monies disproportionate to the amount of service they provided. For example, in 1958 the Beckley Memorial Hospital provided only 20 percent of hospital service in its AMO but consumed 40 percent of the area's funds.[35]

Discussions by administrators concerning the potential for reducing costs at the Memorial Hospitals centered almost exclusively on the underutilization of the hospitals by beneficiaries.[36] On the face of it, this almost myopic focus on occupancy rates at the hospitals is puzzling. Administrators seemed convinced, with very little proof, that costs could be reduced simply through achieving greater economies of scale by increasing the use of the hospitals. However, the attention afforded underutilization probably was motivated more by the concerns of the Fund's trustees instead of by any clear economic rationale. Documents issued by the Fund's Washington office resonate with the desire to meet the trustees' expectations that the hospitals would not merely be kept full, but would be kept full of Fund beneficiaries. Figures 5 and 6 show that with the exception of 1961, the overall occupancy rate of the chain hovered around the 75 percent level for most of the period. Occupancy rates generally were higher at the central hospitals but disturbingly low at some of the community hospitals.

While the contribution of underutilization of the Memorial Hospitals to their high costs cannot be determined precisely, it seems doubtful that costs would have been reduced to acceptable levels even if administrators' efforts to operate the hospitals at capacity had been successful. This conclusion is supported by the experience of Beckley Memorial Hospital. Beckley

Figure 5 Occupancy rate of MMHA hospitals, southern West Virginia and eastern Kentucky, fiscal years 1957–1964

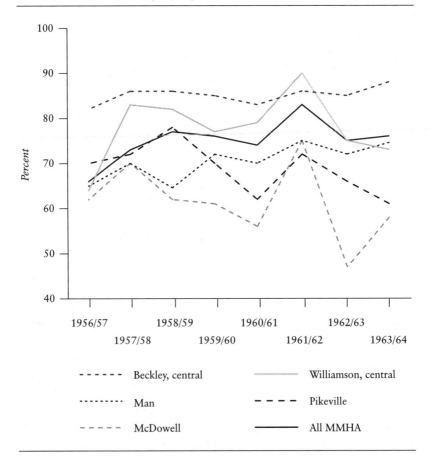

Source: Office of Research and Statistics, "MMHA—Summary Statistics," various years, Fund Archives.

Memorial was the only hospital in the chain to operate at full capacity throughout the life of the MMHA. In fact, a significant additional number of beneficiaries in the Beckley area could have been cared for at Beckley Memorial if more beds had been available.[37] However, despite the fact that the hospital was operating at capacity—and therefore presumably achieving full economies of scale—its costs still remained above the area's average. While the cost per day at Beckley persisted above the $30 level throughout this period, the average charge of other hospitals in the area did not even reach $20 until 1962.[38]

Figure 6 Occupancy rate of MMHA hospitals, southwestern Virginia and southeasterm Kentucky, fiscal years 1957–1964

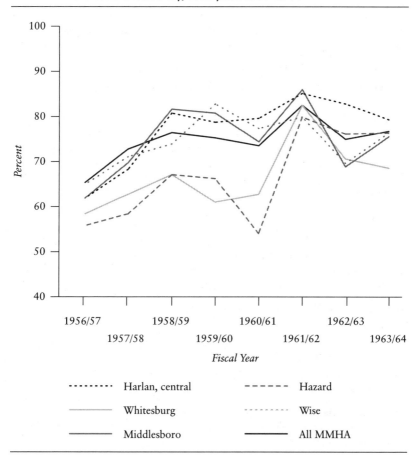

Source: Office of Research and Statistics, "MMHA—Summary Statistics," various years, Fund Archives.

While the Fund's administrators fought a losing battle by attempting to reduce costs at the Memorial Hospitals through increasing occupancy, two familiar phenomena would have caused the continued escalation of costs even if capacity constraints had been met: the level of quality of care in the hospitals and the health needs of the beneficiaries. First, the range of services and the level of care offered by the Memorial Hospitals made them more comparable to metropolitan teaching hospitals than to hospitals in central Appalachia.[39] In fact, the scope of the MMHA's mission was a matter of some debate among Fund administrators. While most administrators argued that the scope of MMHA services should be as broad as possible, others argued that the MMHA was too "luxurious" a set-up, especially since a significant proportion of beneficiaries living outside the service area would not be able to use the hospitals.[40] Perhaps the most vocal detractor within the Fund on this issue was William Riheldaffer, the chief administrator of the Charleston AMO. Encouraging a reevaluation of the MMHA's mission, Riheldaffer stated:

> Continuation of the original concept of the chain idea for hospital operation may have delayed our development of better methods of hospital operation and economies. There is, in my opinion, significant waste of professional and administrative time in supporting a continuation of the chain hospital idea. It is my impression that when these facilities are properly staffed by responsible, dedicated professional and sub-professional personnel they will operate with greater efficiency towards beneficiary service care and increased freedom for all employees of the hospital, at a lower cost.[41]

Even John Newdorp, the MMHA's medical administrator, noted that changes in the provision of care since the initial conception of the chain in 1951 called into question the suitability of the level of care the MMHA was designed to provide. Asked by a reporter whether the Fund had overbuilt hospitals in central Appalachia, Newdorp responded that a "significant" change in the approach to medical care in the intervening years had resulted in a situation where "The active outpatient departments of the hospitals emphasize preventive medicine and early treatment with the result that many patients who might have been hospitalized in the past are now cared for by the doctor in his office instead of being hospitalized."[42] Yet even these reflections about what services the hospitals *should* have provided failed to give appropriate weight to the connection between costs and the level of service they *did* provide. Costs at the Memorial Hospitals would never approach those at competing hospitals as long as the MMHA continued to offer a level of service far above that of its competitors. Even basic indicators suggested that beneficiaries received a different level of care in the Memorial Hospitals. For example, approximately 40 percent of the cases treated in the Beckley Memorial Hospital required surgery, as compared to an average of approximately 26 percent in the area as a whole.[43]

Second, the relatively higher costs of care at the Memorial Hospitals also resulted from the fact that the chain served beneficiaries who were in greater need of medical care than were other members of their communities. This situation was particularly evident at the central hospitals that typically treated more severe cases requiring longer lengths-of-stay. For example, in 1958 the Beckley Memorial Hospital found that 40 percent of its patient base had not received medical treatment in the previous nine years, its psychiatric and physical therapy services—care associated with relatively long lengths-of-stay—operated at capacity, and it cared for a disproportionate number of older and chronically ill patients.[44]

Moreover, the aging of the beneficiary pool was noticeable even within the relatively short life span of the MMHA. Older beneficiaries place greater demands on the health care system in general and on hospitals in particular.[45] Figure 7 shows that beneficiaries over the age of 54 comprised an increasing share of hospital days of care from 1957 until the sale of the MMHA in 1963 and 1964. By 1964, patients over the age of 54 accounted for 47.7 percent of MMHA days of care, up from 42.5 percent in 1957. This shift in beneficiary demographics caused Newdorp to comment in 1961, "The hospitals were planned and located ten years ago. There have been significant changes in the population of the areas they serve. It is very likely that if we were planning this program today, hindsight might change location or size."[46]

In addition to the aging of the beneficiary pool, beneficiaries in central Appalachia placed great demands on the health care system and on hospitals in particular. Central Appalachia had been the most underdeveloped of the coal mining areas before the inception of the Fund with the result that beneficiaries residing in this region suffered disproportionately from neglected medical conditions. In addition, low levels of education and living standards contributed to poor health in this region. Finally, the health needs of the working and retired miners in central Appalachia placed an additional burden on the health care system. Central Appalachia was characterized by high mine injury rates and high rates of respiratory illness produced by mechanization in underground mines.

It is doubtful that the attempt to fill beds in the Memorial Hospitals would have produced cost savings large enough to overcome the costs of

Figure 7   Distribution of hospital days of care by age group,
MMHA hospitals, fiscal years 1957–1964

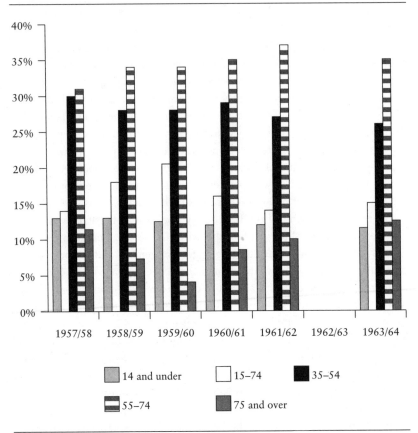

Note: Data from fiscal year 1962/63 are not available

Source: Office of Research and Statistics, "MMHA—Summary Statistics," various years,
Fund Archives.

providing high quality care to a population with above average health
needs. Returning to the experience of the Beckley Memorial Hospital, the
fact that its costs remained significantly above those of its competitors
despite the fact that it operated at capacity was probably due to the combined effects of providing a full range of specialty services to beneficiaries
with a high demand for hospital care.

While administrators focused on increasing occupancy rates to achieve
cost savings, it appears that the trustees were concerned with utilization rates
for other reasons. In this regard, the trustees' insistence on high *beneficiary*

occupancy rates is instructive. Fund beneficiaries as a percentage of all patients in Memorial Hospitals peaked at 84.1 percent in 1958 and then began steadily declining to 72.6 percent by 1961 (the last year for which such data are available). In 1961, three hospitals in southeastern Kentucky— Harlan, Whitesburg, and Middlesboro—could only report less than 62 percent of their occupied beds filled by Fund beneficiaries. Low beneficiary usage looked even more worrisome when combined with low overall utilization rates (see Figures 5 and 6).

The trustees seemed willing to underwrite the relatively high costs of operating the MMHA only as long as beneficiaries were benefiting from its services. From the initial design of the chain little mention was made of expectations regarding costs. Moreover, the Fund had posted operating surpluses of $5.9 million and $7.3 million in the two fiscal years prior to the sale of the chain. Costs were important, certainly, but perhaps not of primary concern to the trustees.

Of greater interest to the trustees was the contribution of beneficiaries' use of the Memorial Hospitals to their attempts to make the hospitals the centerpiece of the Fund. The Memorial Hospitals were part of John L. Lewis's earliest plans to grant miners and their families the highest quality care possible. The hospitals were constructed in order to bring modern facilities, state-of-the-art equipment, and highly trained personnel to beneficiaries in a setting that was undeniably linked to the Fund. The Fund did not simply channel money into local hospitals in order to raise the level of hospital care in the coalfields. The hospitals were at their core a high-profile project designed to increase the significance of the Fund, and by extension the union, in the eyes of the miners. Low utilization of the Memorial Hospitals by beneficiaries diminished the power of this message.

The demise of the MMHA had its roots in the failure of the trustees to see the inherent incompatibility between their vision of the hospitals' mission and the forces unleashed by the new era of industrial relations. The mechanization of the mines accelerated by the 1950 contract reduced the size of beneficiary pool and, therefore, the potential of reaching capacity in the hospitals. Ironically, in 1960 the Fund's trustees would make eligibility cuts in order to rectify the Fund's operating deficits and this action would further reduce the potential hospital population for the MMHA (see chapter 6). In addition, mechanization produced an older and sicker workforce that was perhaps not even best cared for in a hospital setting. Moreover, the Fund's financing mechanism, also a part of the compromise reached in 1950, produced a flow of operating income that was too unstable to meet the needs of operating a chain of hospitals.

The MMHA represented the culmination not only of the administrators' health program, but also of the trustees' political program. The experience of the MMHA provides the best example of the trustees' use of the Fund to achieve political ends, as well as the best example of the insurmountable tensions within that agenda. The Fund's bold experiment in bringing quality hospital care to the coalfields thus became another casualty of the changes in the coal industry unleashed with the blessing by John L. Lewis in 1950.

The Miners Memorial Hospitals epitomized the Fund's managed care program as they incorporated under one roof all the major initiatives that the Fund had promulgated. This point is aptly displayed in the following remarks of Dr. Albert Kistin, the chief of internal medicine at the Beckley Memorial Hospital. Asked why he left a lucrative practice in Washington, D.C., where he was one of the best-known internists in the city, to accept a position at Beckley, Kistin explained:

> I've always dreamed of a chance to work in exactly this kind of medical environment. I really believe the set-up here is terrific. The hospital is organized on a group practice basis—where doctors work as a team, around a core of full-time salaried specialists. Thirty of us are on full-time salary. We don't have to worry about the patient's ability to pay for expensive diagnostic or treatment procedures. We don't have to worry about bills. We can concentrate on giving the best medical service we can. I don't have to worry about making a final diagnosis in a complicated case when I myself am in doubt. I have immediately on call for consultation fine specialists who are practically right at my elbow all the time. The hospital is small enough so that colleagues in other specialties are always within calling distance. You don't have to wait hours, or days, for a consultant to come at his own convenience, often when you're not around, so that he leaves a hastily scrawled note. You can get him at once, and you see the patient together, and talk it over, and pool your opinions on the spot.[47]

The success of the Fund in creating a unique and truly progressive environment for the practice of medicine proved to be a potent recruiting device in attracting physicians like Dr. Kistin to work in underserved areas. The pathbreaking efforts of the MMHA were followed with keen interest by many prominent physicians. When Dr. David Greely, a Harvard graduate and former head of the pediatrics department at Boston University Medical School heard about the construction of the miners' hospitals, he recalled thinking, "'that's the only place for a man with my training.' . . . I wanted to practice in a more challenging place, where I could feel more useful."[48] When he subsequently encountered Dr. McGuiness at a pediatrics conference, he jumped at the offer to serve as chief of clinical services at the Harlan Memorial Hospital.[49]

The MMHA received accolades not only from members of the medical community that shared the Fund's philosophy, but also from other unions, public health professionals, visiting foreign dignitaries, and the media.[50] The hospitals filled a dire need for hospital care in previously neglected areas in a manner that employed an impressive range of innovations designed to keep the quality of care high and the costs of care low. As Deutsch commented, "If it [the MMHA] had made no other contribution, the UMWA Welfare and Retirement Fund would have earned a significant page in American medical history through this trail-blazing act alone. Many medical planners view it as an impressive demonstration of a general pattern that could and should, with modifications based upon regional and economic differences, be adopted widely in the United States."[51] Fund administrators proudly accepted countless awards for their achievements in improving the quality of care available to residents of Appalachia.

The Fund's record of controlling hospital costs through the operation of the MMHA was, however, less clearly effective than its record of improving quality. When the Fund sold the chain in 1963, administrators cited the hospitals' high costs and low beneficiary utilization rates as factors which created an insupportable drain on the Fund's reserves. Facing declining tonnage payments to the Fund as a result of the slump in demand for coal in the late 1950s, the Fund's trustees concluded that, however noble, the effort to provide care in their own hospitals was an expense that the Fund could no longer afford. The experience of the Miners Memorial Hospitals demonstrates the ultimate subordination of the administrators' health policy objectives to the political agenda of the Fund's trustees. The trustees sold the chain because they were only interested in operating the hospitals if they were full of beneficiaries. Chapter 6 will examine the Fund's decision to sell the chain in the context of changes in the fortunes of the coal industry and in the demographics of the beneficiary population.

Yet despite the Memorial Hospitals' relatively short period of operation under the direction of the Fund, their contribution to the development of the health care infrastructure of the coalfields was significant. As with the operation of the retainer program, the development of group practices, and the recruitment of physicians, the Fund's establishment of the MMHA was critical at a time when miners' communities themselves were incapable of providing the stimulus needed for the development of an acceptable and comprehensive system of health care provision. Once the Fund accomplished the difficult task of bringing medical care personnel and facilities to mining communities, it was possible for the communities themselves to undertake the responsibility of sustaining these efforts. In relinquishing control of the Memorial Hospitals, then, the Fund acknowledged its own inability to underwrite such an ambitious program, and also recognized the ability of local communities to support the continuation of services it had helped to establish.

CHAPTER SIX

External Challenges to the Operation of the Fund

*M*any administrators and physicians were drawn to the Fund by the prospect of participating in an experiment that promised to overhaul the provision of care in the coalfields. Administrators and physicians were given free rein to scrutinize all aspects of care; the initiatives they crafted boldly charted new territory in the provision of health services. However, the "experiment" did not take place under carefully controlled conditions, immune to changing circumstances. This chapter describes external factors that significantly affected the Fund's operations: opposition from organized medicine and changes in industry conditions.

Organized medicine roundly denounced the Fund's plans to intervene in the provision of care. Concerned about competition from Fund doctors and hospitals, review of physician decisions by Fund administrators, and the Fund's departure from the lucrative fee-for-service reimbursement system, medical societies from the local to the national level launched a variety of attacks on the Fund's policies. While organized medicine's campaign was not effective everywhere and was largely abandoned by the end of the 1950s, in some places it was potent enough to interfere with the Fund's attempts to recruit physicians and to encourage them to adhere to its practices.

A much more significant challenge to the Fund's operations came from changes in industry conditions in the two decades following the 1950 contract. Two structural changes in the production of coal began their ascendance in the 1950s: the mechanization of underground mines and the increasing use of surface mining. In addition, the industry continued to face intense competition from alternative fuels. These factors—combined with a major downturn in the demand for coal in the late 1950s and early 1960s—contributed to a drastic decline in the number of mines and mining jobs, as well as a decrease in the strength of both the operators and the union.

The changes in industry conditions had ramifications for the operation of the Fund itself, complicating the efforts of administrators to fashion reforms. First, the decline in mining employment generated an aging of the

Fund's beneficiary pool while mechanization increased the hazards faced by underground miners. Hence, changing industry conditions increased the health needs of the Fund's beneficiary pool. Second, the declining prominence of union coal directly affected the Fund's income through the tonnage royalty financing mechanism. The operating deficits and precipitous reduction in reserves that emanated from the downturn in demand threatened the very operation of the Fund.

In the end, the "experiment" that captured the imagination of the Fund's administrators was circumscribed by the same set of forces that brought it into existence. The Fund had been the linchpin in John L. Lewis's truce with the BCOA in 1950. Throughout the next two decades, it was clear that Lewis intended to honor steadfastly the compromise he authored in 1950, regardless of subsequent changes in industry conditions. Eventually, Lewis's actions not only undermined the Fund, but did so in a way that induced the rank-and-file to evaluate critically the stewardship of the union itself.

Opposition from Organized Medicine

As Fund administrators began their reform of the medical care system in the coalfields, they hoped to foster harmonious relations with organized medicine in order to ease the implementation of managed care initiatives. Specifically, the Fund looked to medical societies for help in curtailing abuses like those documented in the Boone Report that were still prevalent in the coalfields. Hopes of cooperation quickly evaporated, however, as Fund administrators encountered stiff opposition to their practices from medical societies at national, state, and local levels. While this opposition generally receded by the end of the 1950s, it had important ramifications for the ability of the Fund to implement its policies in the interim.

The Fund requested the cooperation of organized medicine on two fronts: in rectifying violations of medical ethics and in promoting congenial relations between the Fund and medical societies. First, the Fund asked local medical societies to deal with carefully documented instances of unacceptable physician behavior. Fund administrators themselves were uncomfortable with the role of "fingering" incompetent physicians. Moreover, it was purportedly the duty of medical societies to prevent their members from performing services for which they lacked qualifications and from engaging in unethical treatment and billing practices. In 1952, to convince organized medicine of the need for such actions, Warren Draper encouraged the AMA to send a survey team to areas the Fund identified as particularly in need of attention. In reporting its results, the survey team confirmed Draper's assertion that abuses that endangered the quality of health care persisted unchecked throughout the coal fields.[1]

Second, the Fund asked for organized medicine's cooperation in building harmonious relations among medical societies, Fund administrators, and physicians. Fund administrators wanted to create an environment that would be most conducive to achieving their objectives. Specifically, the Fund needed physicians to serve beneficiaries, and to serve them in a manner that conformed to its treatment, billing, and review practices. Opposition from organized medicine to these practices would, in the Fund's estimation, adversely affect its ability to reform a system of care which otherwise produced overutilization and excessive charges.

Much to their dismay, Fund administrators soon discovered that organized medicine would act more as an impediment to reform than as a partner in their plans for progress. For most of the 1950s, organized medicine viewed the Fund with suspicion. Local physicians feared that the Fund would promote competition that would undermine their practices. One physician called members of a group practice "a bunch of young punks come out here to try [to] cut into my $30,000 a year practice."[2] Fears of competition were greatest in areas suffering from the depression in the coal markets. In regions hit hard by the decline in the demand for coal, the Fund provided a valuable source of guaranteed income for participating physicians. Local physicians were afraid that the Fund's participating physicians list would prevent them from treating Fund beneficiaries at a time when private resources for medical care in the communities were scarce.[3]

Organized medicine also cast a wary eye on the Fund's practice of examining physicians' decisions. Unimpressed by administrators' review of treatment and billing, one physician referred to the Fund as a "dictatorship."[4] Furthermore, an AMA report noted that physicians discerned a potential for additional undesirable regulations: "These fears are not founded upon tangible, definite actions or any innovation in the UMWA plans, but are due to the apprehension that some new Union rule or regulation might develop which might curtail their opportunities to continue to provide service to mine workers who, in many instances, comprise the greater part of their practices."[5] Organized medicine, in short, did not share health experts' enthusiasm for the Fund's innovations. Rather, medical societies concluded that the Fund posed a threat to their previously unassailable ability to dictate health policy.

Before any of its fears were actually realized, organized medicine attacked the Fund from both the national and local level. First, on the national level, the AMA repeatedly stated its opposition to any Fund policies that interfered with physician autonomy and patients' right to choose their physician. After sponsoring four conferences between 1952 and 1956 that examined the provision of medical care in the coalfields, in 1957 the AMA appointed a committee to specify procedures for dealing with the Fund. Consistent with recommendations of the previous conferences, the committee insisted upon fee-for-service reimbursement, unrestricted choice of doctors, and the elimination of review of physician services. In addition, the AMA took its campaign to a broader audience through a public relations blitz—receiving attention in *Fortune* and *Life*—on the advantages of freedom of choice of physicians.[6]

The most significant point of conflict on the national level came in 1955 when Draper announced the Fund's intention to institute a preadmission consultation policy. Designed to prevent unqualified physicians from performing surgery, the policy required physicians to receive authorization for hospitalization from an approved specialist or from the Fund. Organized medicine vehemently opposed this attempt by the Fund to circumscribe physician behavior. The magnitude of the conflict eventually forced Draper to withdraw the requirement.[7]

The AMA's stance also fueled potent actions by local medical societies. First, the AMA did not provide leadership in the drive to compel local societies to police their members as requested by the Fund. As a result, local medical societies rarely penalized in a substantive fashion even the most flagrant infractions of medical ethics by their members. As a Fund administrator noted:

> Physicians are particularly loathe to sit in judgement of their fellows and discipline them. Regardless of the extensive literature emanating from headquarters of out various medical organizations stressing the need of the medical profession to clean their own dirty linen, hospital staffs, city and county medical societies, act only in very rare cases to force its members who are not in line with the high ethical standards of the profession to reform.[8]

For instance, when a state medical society found a physician guilty of fee splitting and ghost surgery, it disciplined him with a 24-hour, secret suspension. The punishment seemed even more inadequate in light of other aspects of the physician's record: 75 percent of the appendectomies he performed were found to be unnecessary, and his failure to keep his records up to date resulted in the failure of a local hospital to receive accreditation.[9]

Second, local medical societies often worked to bar members of group practices affiliated with the Fund from obtaining hospital privileges. For example, an obstetrician-gynecologist working at the Bellaire Clinic could not get admitting privileges in a local hospital, despite the fact that he was the county's only board-certified obstetrician-gynecologist.[10] All of the Russellton Clinic's doctors were denied admitting privileges at the two local hospitals, forcing them to treat their patients at hospitals in Pittsburgh.[11] Similarly, local physicians often refused to refer their patients to MMHA hospitals, charging that the hospitals competed unfairly with other local hospitals.[12]

The hostile atmosphere engendered by the friction between the Fund and local medical societies affected the Fund's ability to recruit and retain physicians, and to encourage physicians to conform to its policies. The unpleasant tenor of the conflict had particularly acute effects in the small communities where most of the physicians affiliated with the Fund served. Reflecting on the psychological effects of local medical societies' opposition to the Fund, Warren Draper noted in an address at the AMA annual meeting in 1959, "Many of these physicians have suffered abuse and criticism and have been hampered in their work by less understanding colleagues, because they believed in the fund's objectives and continued to serve its beneficiaries, without regard to controversial issues and with a desire only to help their fellow man."[13] The fact that many Fund physicians were denied membership in local medical societies only added insult to injury.[14]

As the 1950s progressed, tensions between the Fund and organized medicine increased despite efforts on both sides to fashion a truce. However, toward the end of the decade organized medicine began to rethink its position. First, medical societies' opposition to Fund policies had been based largely on the *potential* for destructive competition, oppressive review, and a general decrease in physician fees. As Fund operations unfolded, however, few of these eventualities were realized. For example, in 1956 a member of AMA's survey team assessed the situation in Bluefield and Beckley,

> [local physicians] admitted without qualification that they recognized a definite need for more hospital beds in this area. Further, the existing medical agencies have not been adversely affected by the opening of the Beckley Memorial Hospital. The physicians themselves, with only one exception, also admitted that they were financially in no way harmed by the opening of this new hospital. In some instances, physicians admitted that their income had increased.[15]

These views were echoed by a physician with a private practice in the Beckley area,

> I suppose we were all a bit jittery, and some of us angry, when they first started to build that hospital. We were concerned that it might prove a serious economic competitor, and take our patients away from us. As it turned out, there was plenty of doctoring business for all, and most of us are better off. Specialists among us get paid by the UMWA Fund for needed home and office treatment of its beneficiaries. In these hard times, when large numbers of jobless miners haven't enough to pay medical bills for themselves or their families, it means a lot.[16]

Physicians in many areas realized that the Fund's ability to provide needed reimbursement for the care of miners—working, retired, and unemployed—and their families was more crucial than its unorthodox policies.

Second, by increasing the supply of quality care, the Fund had developed a reputation that spoke for itself. In view of the Fund's achievements, organized medicine's claims that the Fund's policies jeopardized the provision of medical care and the rights of the patient simply were unconvincing. Miners and their families stuck by the Fund and were not swayed by organized medicine's appeals for "freedom of choice." Henry Schmidt, the president of North American Coal and the operators' trustee for the Fund backed up administrators' policies:

> The Fund has every right to insist that its miner-beneficiaries should not be exposed to substandard medicine. When it set up standards of quality that are applicable to all physicians and hospitals, it is not interfering with the patient's right of free choice. The Fund has every moral and economic right to drop doctors or hospitals from its approved list when they fail to meet those minimum standards. I support Mr. Lewis 100% on this position. I have every confidence in Dr. Draper, whose distinguished record in medicine speaks for itself. When he tells me that a doctor or a hospital does not meet Fund qualifications for good medical care, I will accept his word without question.[17]

Finally, physicians in some areas of the coalfields attested to the benefits of working with the Fund. As a physician with a private practice in the Beckley area stated, "The staff doctors at the hospital do good medicine, and, with few exceptions, they and we get along well. Our county medical society is open to them, and most of them belong to it. I must say, on the whole, that medical standards in this community have been raised by having the hospital doctors in it."[18]

Thus, miners, employers and even a significant number of local physicians were unmoved by organized medicine's criticisms of the Fund. Moreover, the reaction of medical societies was beginning to compare unfavorably to that of Fund administrators, as suggested by the comments of a physician treating Fund beneficiaries:

> I have followed fairly closely the difficulties which have developed between the Area Medical Office and certain medical societies in western Pennsylvania, and some parts of West Virginia and Ohio. I would like to go on record as saying that I feel that many of these societies or at least some very vociferous groups have in many instances acted without mature thought or without basis for the positions they have taken. In contrast, I am inclined to think that the Area Medical Office has spoken with considerable restraint and that the decisions which you have reached seem to me to be the most equitable in the great majority of instances.[19]

As time wore on, organized medicine's campaign against the Fund appeared to be playing to a smaller and smaller audience.

Warren Draper, capitalizing on a reputation earned within the AMA, eloquently defended the Fund's position to its remaining opponents by standing organized medicine's appeal for "freedom of choice" on its head. In an address at the AMA annual meeting in 1959 (reprinted in the *Journal of the American Medical Association*), Draper contended that the phrase "freedom of choice" was easily appropriable by groups eager to secure a "rallying cry to awaken an emotional response without understanding or recognizing the facts." He noted that before the advent of the Fund, miners and their families had virtually no choice of physician. By contrast, the Fund reimbursed a wide range of physicians, granting beneficiaries access to a number of providers—including specialists and distant medical centers—who previously would not have treated them. He concluded, "It would seem that, by increasing the free choice of physicians to many thousands, and by placing no limit on the extent to which the highest quality of service will be provided, the UMWA welfare and retirement fund has qualified under terms of fairness and justice as a leading collaborator in recognizing the value and expanding the scope of free choice of physician."[20] A careful reading of Draper's remarks reveals the fundamental hypocrisy of organized medicine's stated position: it demanded unrestricted freedom of choice of physicians only when it suited the interests of its members. Draper stopped short of explicitly noting that organized medicine never condemned the complete lack of choice of physician inherent in the company doctor system.

Organized medicine was, in fact, much more troubled by encroachment by third parties like the Fund on physician autonomy than it was with patients' freedom of choice.

Unfounded fears combined with the Fund's growing reputation made organized medicine's claims look increasingly spurious. Therefore, in June 1959, the AMA House of Delegates officially retreated from its criticism of the Fund by qualifying its call for "freedom of choice" of physicians with the phrases "wherever practicable" and "universally as practicable."[21] While a few local medical societies, most notably those in the areas served by the Bellaire and Russellton Clinics, continued to oppose the Fund's practices, in general, opposition from organized medicine decreased in the 1960s. It appeared that the Fund had largely overcome what an AMA report identified as its "greatest problem:" "overcoming the fears and uncertainties of the medical profession facing a new form of practice."[22] However, it is important to note that while the Fund ultimately was victorious in its struggle to cultivate peaceful, if uneasy, relations with organized medicine, administrators found that this struggle hindered their implementation of managed care policies throughout the 1950s.

Changes in Industry Conditions

Three major events in the 1950s redefined the positions of the unionized coal operators and the UMWA: mechanization, increased competition from strip mining, and a fall in the demand for coal. Together these events spawned a shake-out of firms and workers alike as the industry became more concentrated and the number of mines and miners decreased. This maturation of the coal industry had important ramifications for the operation of the Fund itself.

The large operators and John L. Lewis instigated the first major change in the coal industry when they agreed to mechanize the mines in 1950. The replacement of hand-loading with machine cutting and loading of coal in underground mines nearly doubled productivity by the end of the decade: average short tons per miner-day increased from 5.75 in 1950 to 10.64 in 1960.[23] However, mechanization was not introduced in all mines. Small mine owners generally were unable to make the capital investments necessary to mechanize and, furthermore, tended to mine marginal veins that were less suitable for mechanized mining techniques. Unable to reap the savings in labor costs generated by mechanization, many small mines were forced either to operate nonunion or to go out of business altogether.[24]

Second, surface mining, a relatively new method of mining, gained prominence in the postwar period. In 1940, surface mining accounted for less than 10 percent of all coal mined in the United States.[25] By 1950, however, its rapidly rising popularity was clear as surface mining produced 23.9 percent of all coal that year (see Figure 8). A decade later, surface mining claimed 31.4 percent of all coal and by 1972, surface mining would surpass underground mining as the leading mining method. It should be noted, however, that given the relatively greater labor intensity of underground mining, the bulk of the mining workforce continued to labor underground (see Figure 9).

There were important regional differences in the use of surface mining. Specifically, surface mining was far more prevalent in the coalfields west of

Figure 8   Coal production by mining method, 1950–1979

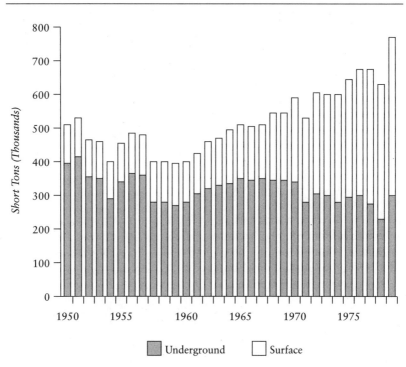

Source: U.S. Department of Labor, Bureau of Labor Statistics, *Technology, Production, and Labor in the Bituminous-Coal Industry, 1950–79,* by Rose N. Zeisel et al., Bulletin 2072 (Washington, D.C.: GPO, 1981): Table 8, 13.

Figure 9   Employment by mining method, 1950–1979

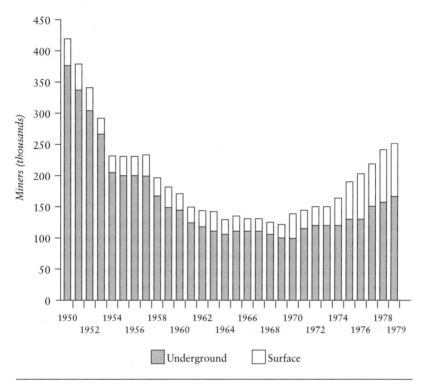

Source: U.S. Department of Labor, Bureau of Labor Statistics, Table 28, 39.

Appalachia. In 1950, 10 percent of Appalachian miners worked in surface mines, 30 percent of interior miners worked in surface mines, and 15 percent of western miners worked in surface mines. By 1975, regional differences were even more prominent as 25 percent of Appalachian miners worked in surface mines, 47 percent of interior miners worked in surface mines, and 55 percent of western miners worked in surface mines. In absolute terms, however, Appalachia employed the vast majority of the mining workforce; from 1950 to 1975, between 85 and 90 percent of all underground miners and 65 to 75 percent of all surface miners worked in Appalachia.[26]

Third, with the exception of a brief recovery in the middle of the decade, the demand for coal decreased throughout the 1950s and remained particularly sluggish from 1958 to 1962 (see Figure 8). Most of the decline can be attributed to continuing competition from oil and natural gas. The ability of alternative fuels to whittle away coal's share of the energy market was proving to be a nettlesome problem. After all, the reorganization of the industry in 1950 had, in large part, been in response to competition from oil and gas and, yet, coal's competitiveness still lagged. In 1950 coal had been only narrowly edged out by oil as the country's leading energy source: coal comprised 38.3 percent of energy consumption while oil constituted 39.6 percent of the energy market and gas trailed in third place with only 17.8 percent of the energy market. By 1960, coal's significance as an energy source had diminished markedly: coal comprised only 23.0 percent of energy consumption, roughly half of oil's 45.3 percent market share and behind even gas with 28.1 percent of the market.[27]

Together, mechanization, the increasingly prevalence of surface mining, and the decline in the demand for coal affected coal operators disparately; the magnitude of the impact of industry conditions depended on the size of mining operations. Overall, the industry appeared to be in considerable distress. In 1960, the net income of coal mining firms after taxes was a mere 0.5 percent of their net worth, far below the 6.4 percent registered by manufacturing firms.[28] However, these aggregate figures mask the fact that the largest coal companies continued to be profitable. The elimination of small mines and a wave of mergers served to increase the concentration of the coal industry in the 1950s. In 1950 the eight largest coal operators had produced 19 percent of the total industry output while by 1960, these eight firms produced 33 percent of total industry output.[29] By 1973, 4,779 mines would be eliminated from the industry.[30] The larger firms that emerged during this period—those most closely linked to the BCOA—were better able to weather the demand slump than the aggregate figures would suggest. For example, Consolidation Coal and Eastern Associated showed net profits of $12 million and $3 million respectively in 1955. In 1960, in the midst of the demand slump, their profits had almost doubled—to $21 million for Consolidation Coal (a 6.7 percent return) and $5 million for Eastern Associated (a 4.5 percent return). Five years later, their earnings continued to rise as Consolidation Coal posted $34 million in profits (an 8.7 percent return) and Eastern Associated reported $9 million in profits (a 13.2 percent return).[31]

The changes in industry conditions also affected the position of the UMWA, most notably through the decrease in mining employment. Mechanization and the drop in demand prompted operators to trim their workforces. In one decade, employment in coal mines fell 59 percent from

415,600 miners in 1950 to 169,400 miners in 1960 (see Figure 9). While employment would continue to fall until the early 1970s, the bulk of the layoffs occurred in the 1950s.

The Union's position was not only influenced by the general decrease in the number of jobs in coal mining, but also by the increasing prominence of surface mining operations. The rise of surface mining was a matter of concern to the UMWA since surface mines were less likely to be unionized than underground mines.[32] While both surface and underground workforces were reduced during the 1950s and 1960s, the surface mining workforce fell only 11.7 percent from 1955 to 1965, comparatively less than the 44.5 percent reduction in the underground workforce. This difference served to alter the composition of the mining workforce overall: in 1955, 12.1 percent of the mining workforce worked in surface mines; a decade later 17.9 percent worked in surface mines, and by 1975, 28.9 percent of miners would work in surface mines.

As the prominence of coal as an energy source declined, so too did the UMWA's strength. Its ability to disrupt production, its major source of power in the 1940s, became increasingly less potent as coal users were better able to switch to alternative fuels or to purchase coal from nonunion suppliers. From 1947 to 1959, the percentage of nonunion coal increased from 10.0 percent to 35.8 percent of all coal production. By 1968 union coal had regained some of its market share, but nonunion coal still produced a quarter of all coal in the United States.[33] In addition, by the late 1960s, the UMWA represented only 75 to 80 percent of coal miners,[34] a decline from standard estimates that placed union representation at above 90 percent of all miners in the 1940s.

The changes in the industry conditions would have a considerable impact on the operations of the Fund. The 1950s and 1960s witnessed alterations in the size and composition of the Fund's beneficiary pool as well as a perilous decline in the Fund's income. The diminishing strength of both the signatory operators and the union, combined with the requirements of the pact they had formed in 1950, would circumscribe the options available to shield the Fund's operations from the changes in the industry.

Changes in the Fund's Beneficiary Pool

Any discussion of changes in the nature of the Fund's beneficiary pool must begin with a few important observations about the prevailing level of health in mining communities when the Fund began operations in the late 1940s.

Fund administrators faced a formidable challenge in caring for a population whose health needs had been largely neglected prior to the inception of the Fund's operations. A miner's life expectancy in 1947 was only 56 years, well below the U.S. average of 66 years.[35] Mining was a dangerous occupation which carried with it high rates of injury and illness. The conditions in mining towns, as documented in the Boone Report, further compromised the health of the mining population. Rudimentary sanitation, poor diets, and low levels of education increased the prevalence of disease and early death in the coal camps.

It should be noted, however, that the health status of miners and their families did vary somewhat by their proximity to urban areas and by their type of employer. Mining families who lived within reasonable distances to urban areas and had access to adequate transportation routes to those areas, were more likely to have access to quality health care providers. In addition, as in the past, miners who worked for large, captive mines typically enjoyed safer working conditions, lived in better camps, and were provided with better health care than their counterparts in smaller mines.

Mechanization heightened the health needs of the Fund's beneficiary pool through its impact on the size and composition of the workforce, and through its impact on the hazards faced by working miners. First, the changes in industry conditions that allowed operators to trim their workforces altered the age profile of the beneficiary pool. As fewer positions became available in the mines, the workforce not only became smaller, but it also became older as fewer younger workers obtained employment.[36] The fact that the Fund continued to cover miners after they retired further magnified the aging of the beneficiary pool.

While the Fund did not collect data on the ages of all its beneficiaries, it did note the ages of those using its hospital services. The median age of beneficiaries admitted to hospitals climbed steadily from 37.8 years in 1953 to 54.3 years in 1966.[37] Figure 10 shows the distribution of hospital services by age group from 1953 to 1965. The impact of the aging of the mining population is seen in the decline in the proportion of hospital services used by younger beneficiaries and the concomitant increase in the proportion of services used by older ones.

The aging of the mining population also displays regional variation. Figures 11 and 12 show the median age of beneficiaries admitted to hospitals in each AMO from 1953 to 1965.[38] These figures demonstrate that the central Appalachian areas in Figure 11—Charleston, Beckley, Louisville, and Knoxville—had relatively younger beneficiary pools than the remaining

Figure 10   Distribution of all Fund hospital discharges by age group, 1953–1965

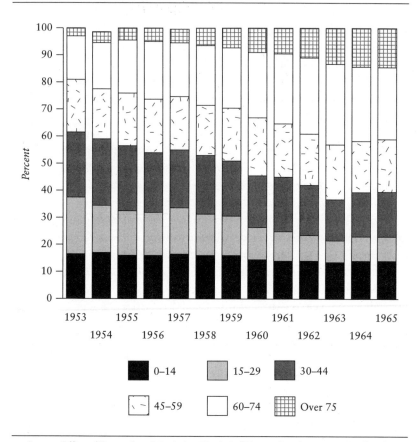

Source: Office of Research and Statistics, "Statistical Report," various years, Fund Archives.

coalfield areas featured in Figure 12. This regional pattern is motivated, in part, by the predominance of the relatively more arduous underground mining in central Appalachia requiring a younger workforce. Again, despite this regional variation, it should be noted that the beneficiary pools in each area show a consistent aging over time.

Second, in addition to altering the composition of the beneficiary pool, mechanization increased the occupational hazards faced by miners working in underground mines. In eliminating the strenuous task of cutting and loading coal by hand, the machines heightened the level of dust and noise in the mines. Elevated dust and noise levels increased the two major sources of health hazards in underground mines: roof falls that produce injuries and

Figure 11 Median age of Fund beneficiaries admitted to hospitals, central Appalachian Areas, 1953–1966

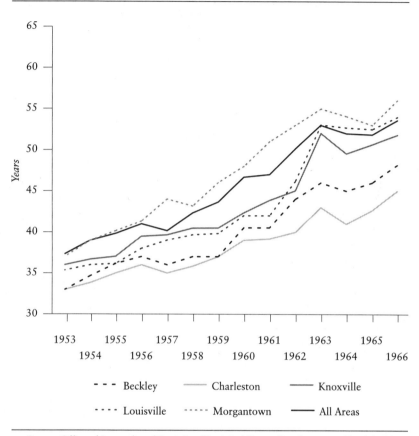

Source: Office of Research and Statistics, "Statistical Report," various years, Fund Archives.

dust levels that produce respiratory illnesses. While mechanization reduced the injuries associated with the cutting and lifting heavy loads of coal, it increased the injuries associated with roof falls as the noise produced by the machines diminished miners' ability to listen for stresses in the roofs. As a result, the injury rate did not decrease between 1950 and 1970.[39] The fatality rate actually increased in this period; in 1946 there were 1.08 fatalities per million hours worked, in 1960 the fatality rate rose to 1.13, and by 1968 the rate had reached a post-war high of 1.37 fatalities per million hours worked.[40]

Mechanization also raised the level of dust in underground mines, thereby greatly increasing the incidence of illnesses associated with the

Figure 12　Median age of Fund beneficiaries admitted to hospitals, northern and southern Appalachia, interior and western Areas, 1953–1966

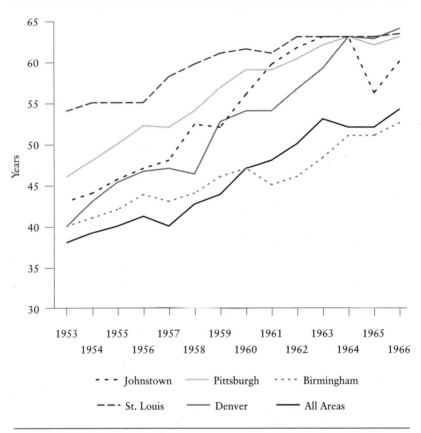

Source: Office of Research and Statistics, "Statistical Report," various years, Fund Archives.

inhalation of dust, commonly referred to as "black lung disease."[41] Hence, miners who managed to retain their jobs as mechanization proceeded were in greater danger of developing ailments that required substantial medical attention. It should be noted, however, that mechanization's effect on the prevalence of black lung was not immediately discernable to miners and their physicians. Slow recognition was due, in part, to the fact that black lung typically takes a number of years to develop to a stage where it can be diagnosed as a mining-related disease. More importantly, the UMWA leadership turned a blind eye to identifying the causes of black lung until the 1970s (see below) with the result that its links to mechanization were not fully understood until a generation of miners had been disabled by the disease.

Surface mining remained relatively safer than underground mining. Surface miners still faced the above-average workplace hazards associated with outdoor work and work with heavy equipment, but they experienced far lower rates of injury and illness compared to underground miners. The non-fatal disabling injury rate in surface mines has been less than half the rate in underground mines since World War II and has fallen throughout most of the postwar period. Moreover, injuries in surface mines tend to be less severe than those in underground mines.[42] The prevalence of respiratory diseases associated with mining is also lower in surface mines: in 1975 the National Institute for Occupational Safety and Health estimated that only 2.5 percent of surface miners suffered from coal workers' pneumoconiosis (cwp) while 13.0 percent of working underground miners suffered from cwp.[43]

In summary, changes in coal production technologies had important implications for the health needs of the Fund's beneficiaries. The improvements in productivity furnished by mechanization and surface mining reduced job growth in the industry and, consequently, resulted in a steady aging of the Fund's beneficiary pool. Since mechanization also increased the occupational hazards in underground mines, those miners who managed to survive the layoffs of the 1950s eventually would place increasing demands on the health care system. Therefore, changes in industry conditions served to increase the difficulties Fund administrators faced in caring for miners and their families. In addition to overcoming the legacy of a history of inferior medical care in the coalfields, administrators also were required to provide for an aging and progressively sicker population.

Addressing the Decline in the Fund's Income

The decline in the demand for coal directly affected the Fund's income through the tonnage royalty financing mechanism. Figure 13 shows the income received by the Fund from the 40-cent tonnage royalty in effect from 1952 to 1971. The downturn in coal production in the late 1950s resulted in a decrease in royalty payments to the Fund. In fact, as shown in Table 13, the drop in royalties was proportionately greater than the fall in coal production. During the downturn from 1957 to 1961, coal production fell 22.0 percent while tonnage royalties fell 26.3 percent. This outcome was due partly to the fact that union coal declined as percentage of all coal mined throughout the postwar period. In addition, the proportionately greater decline in royalty payments resulted from the existence of "sweetheart contracts" between local unions and signatory mines facing financial hardship. Local unions often agreed to overlook their employers' delinquency in making payments to the Fund in order to keep the mines in operation as union mines. This practice was particularly prevalent in regions hardest hit by the industry's downturn: eastern Kentucky, Virginia, and parts of West Virginia.[44]

The decline in income had severe consequences for the financial health of the Fund. As shown in Figure 14, in 1959 the Fund spent more than it received for the first time since 1953. The 1959 deficit of $11.3 million grew 62 percent over the next year to $18.3 million, and remained high at $16.5 million in 1961. The deficits were caused primarily by the reduction in royalty income as the Fund's total expenditures remained fairly stable in the late 1950s (see Figure 15). As a result of its declining income and oper-

Figure 13 Tonnage royalty payments received by the Fund, 1952–1971

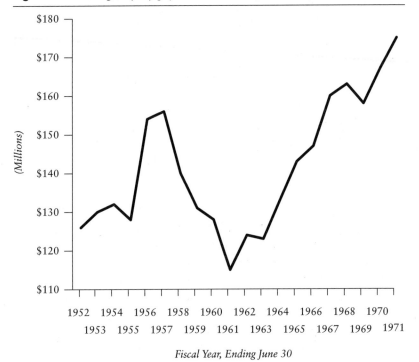

Fiscal Year, Ending June 30

Source: UMWA Welfare and Retirement Fund, *Annual Report,* various years.

ating deficits, the Fund's reserves began dropping precipitously after a five-year period of sustained growth (see Figure 16). In the period from 1959 to 1962, reserves fell 31.6 percent from $145.8 million to $99.8 million.

The precarious state of the Fund's finances caused considerable concern among its trustees, John L. Lewis, Josephine Roche, and Henry Schmidt. Lewis's continued adherence to the 1950 compromise with the large operators prevented him from proposing increases in operator contributions to the Fund (see below). The trustees' concerns over the Fund's finances were not allayed by Fund administrators' conviction that the managed care reforms they introduced in the 1950s would render cost savings. The trustees realized that any cost savings that arose from managed care—in the

Table 13 Coal production (thousand short tons) and amount of coal production contributing royalty payments to the Fund, 1952–1971

Fiscal Year	Total Production	Tonnage Producing Royalties	Royalty Tonnage as a % of Total Production
1952	511,378	314,337	61.5%
1953	450,060	324,226	72.0
1954	416,014	330,922	79.5
1955	423,253	319,800	75.6
1956	502,893	382,215	76.0
1957	499,099	388,297	77.8
1958	440,128	345,744	78.6
1959	424,003	327,453	77.2
1960	415,041	318,954	76.8
1961	389,216	286,231	73.5
1962	428,912	309,013	72.0
1963	431,450	308,028	71.4
1964	470,780	333,717	70.9
1965	496,519	356,562	71.8
1966	519,794	366,234	70.5
1967	560,769	399,622	71.3
1968	550,543	407,724	74.1
1969	544,207	393,702	72.3
1970	580,035	416,637	71.8
1971	614,987	436,735	71.0

Note: The percentage of coal that contributed royalty payments is only an imperfect measure of the extent of union production as the UMWA allowed some union operators to defer or even neglect to pay royalties.

Sources: Total production figures for the fiscal year are compiled from monthly coal production reported in the U.S. Department of the Interior, Bureau of Mines, *Minerals Yearbook*. Production contributing royalties is derived by dividing royalty payments received by the 40 cent royalty rate. Royalty payments are reported in UMWA Welfare and Retirement Fund, *Annual Report*.

Figure 14   Fund receipts less Fund expenditures, 1952–1971

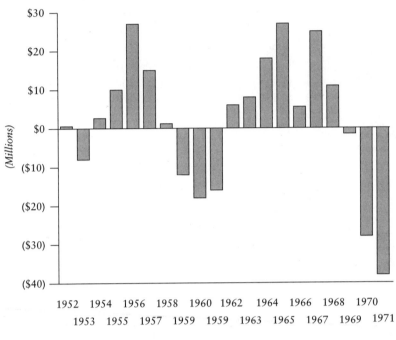

Fiscal Year, Ending June 30

Source: UMWA Welfare and Retirement Fund, *Annual Report.*

form of reduced hospitalization, a decrease in the amount of unnecessary treatment, and a decline in excessive charges—would only be evident in the long term. Unwilling to endure operating deficits in the interim, the trustees refused to rely solely on managed care initiatives to produce cost savings.

Managed care initiatives also were ill-suited to the trustees' objectives since their implementation lagged behind the appearance of high costs. Many of the managed care reforms were not even in place when the trustees sought to redress the Fund's first operating deficit in 1953. Moreover, the severe drop in income in the late 1950s and early 1960s occurred just as Fund administrators were implementing some of their most ambitious managed care reforms. Most notably, the operation of the MMHA hospitals from 1956 to 1963 coincided with the Fund's lowest ever intake of royalty payments.

While unconvinced about managed care's ability to reduce costs, the trustees largely rejected proposals to reduce the Fund's costs by restricting

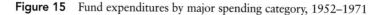

Figure 15   Fund expenditures by major spending category, 1952–1971

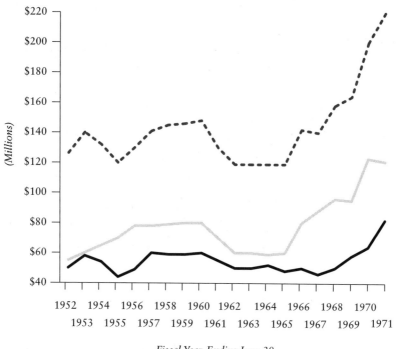

Fiscal Year, Ending June 30

- - - - - Total Expenditures   Pensions   Health

Source: UMWA Welfare and Retirement Fund, *Annual Report.*

the scope of services provided by the plan. Fund administrators opposed cutting services on the grounds that such eliminations would only increase costs elsewhere.[45] For example, placing a cap on the number of hospital days covered by the Fund would encourage patients to leave the hospital when their coverage expired, instead of when their medical conditions warranted discharge. In such cases, patients might not recover adequately with the result that further hospitalization would be needed at additional expense to the Fund.

Instead, the trustees concentrated on reducing expenditures in order to eliminate the Fund's operating deficits. The trustees attained cost savings through two drastic actions: reducing the size of the beneficiary pool and

Figure 16   Unexpended balance (reserves) of the Fund, 1952–1971

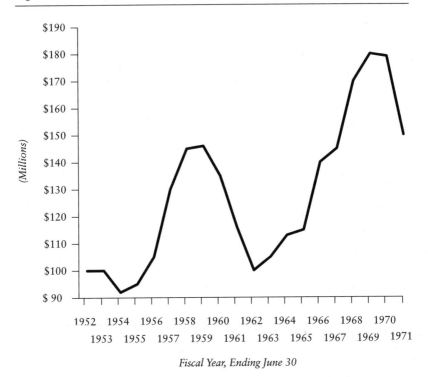

Fiscal Year, Ending June 30

Source: UMWA Welfare and Retirement Fund, *Annual Report.*

selling the Miners Memorial Hospitals. The primary cost-cutting strategy was the reduction of the size of the beneficiary pool. This approach was consistent with the philosophy John L. Lewis had espoused in agreeing to the mechanization of the mines. A decline in employment, Lewis argued, was an acceptable cost for the union to bear in exchange for an improvement in the position of miners who retained their jobs. Tightening eligibility standards for Fund programs embodied essentially the same spirit: the union would provide premium care, but only for a select portion of the mining population. The trustees were also careful, whenever possible, to trim the most marginal beneficiaries from the Fund's rolls in order to preserve the returns to loyalty that accrued from the union's provision of benefits.

The trustees first cut eligibility for Fund services in 1953 when they restricted the supply of pensions to those miners who had accrued the requisite 20 years of service within the 30 years prior to their retirement.[46]

This ruling affected many miners who had fought to build the union during difficult times and had become disabled during their forties and fifties, eleven or more years prior to their retirement. For example, Odell Gwynn was a West Virginia miner who had spent 28 years in the mines and was denied a pension as a result of this policy. He had entered the mines at age 15 and was one of the first miners to sign a union card during the organizing drives of the 1930s. Gwynn had served as vice-president of his local and had participated in the 1946 strike which lead to the formation of the Fund. In 1949, at the age of 43, Gwynn suffered an injury in the mines that prevented him from returning to work. When he reached retirement age in 1965, Gwynn was declared ineligible for a pension under the 1953 rules. Despite his long years of service—during critical moments in the UMWA's history—Gwynn was denied his pension because he had not accumulated 20 years of service within the 30-year period before his retirement.[47]

A year after the changes to the pension rules, the trustees voted to stop monthly benefit payments to 30,000 disabled miners and 24,000 widows.[48] The Fund had been providing modest monthly stipends to widows and disabled miners who were ineligible for pensions or for Social Security and were otherwise destitute. Disturbed by the $7.5 million operating deficit of the previous year, the trustees claimed that the costs of caring for disabled miners, and widows and their dependents for indefinite periods was simply too high. The Fund saved roughly $8 million by reducing its outlays for widows and their dependents,[49] and approximately $4 million to $9 million by eliminating monthly payments to disabled miners.[50] Moreover, the trustees claimed that the burden of such care should fall on the state.[51]

The eligibility cuts in 1953 and 1954 affected some of the most marginal and needy segments of the mining population. The trustees actions received particularly vocal criticism from Allen Croyle, secretary of Local 3648 in St. Michael, Pennsylvania,

> Never did March winds blow with such chilling for this cruel act strikes a foul blow to the economic vitals of these unfortunate people. The Trustees calloused disregard for the tragic plight of the widows and orphans, the crippled, the maimed and the sick, strikes us with a suffocating sense of woe. These people are doomed to the indignity of a life on relief or become a galling burden to their families.[52]

The trustees' actions severed one of the few sources of income available to the elderly, the sick, and the widowed. For instance, disability payments were one of the only avenues of aid available to miners ineligible for pensions because they had retired before May 28, 1946.[53] These were the miners who had been featured so prominently in the Boone Report. However poignant the plight of these groups, they contributed little in economic terms to the union: they did not work, they were not expected to work again, and they did not pay dues. Consequently, widows and disabled miners fell victim to the cold calculus of trustees bent on reducing costs that were not accompanied by sufficient countervailing benefits.

The trustees' most drastic eligibility cutbacks came in the early 1960s as they attempted to eliminate the operating losses spawned by the industry's recession. In mid-1960 the trustees revoked medical care for all miners unemployed for a year or more, for union miners whose employers refused to sign national wage agreements, and for those miners who operated their own mines.[54] A total of 40,729 beneficiaries lost their health benefits as a result of the policy change, over 94 percent of whom had been unemployed for a year or more.[55] Overall, 17.7 percent of Fund beneficiaries had their health coverage canceled. Cancellations were severest in central Appalachia where unemployment was particularly high and where miners and their families were probably most in need of Fund support. Also in 1960, the trustees reduced pensions from $100 to $75 per month. Finally, in 1962 the trustees eliminated coverage for miners whose employers were behind in their royalty payments.[56]

The eligibility cuts reduced expenditures significantly in the period between fiscal years 1960 and 1962 and, for the following three years, allowed expenditures to remain at levels below those posted in the 1950s (see Figure 15). Once income began to grow after the coal markets recovered beginning in 1961, the Fund was able to report operating surpluses and a steady increase in its reserves throughout the remainder of the decade (see Figures 13, 14 and 16).

The improved financial health of the Fund lead the trustees to alter some of their decisions concerning pension rules. In 1965 the trustees raised pensions twice, first to $85 and then to $100; lowered the retirement age to 55; and mandated that a miner's final year of service be in a union mine in order to receive a pension.[57] The trustees' actions again exposed their preoccupation with enhancing the competitive position of large mine owners. Specifically, encouraging miners to retire diminished the supply of labor available to nonunion mines.[58] The stipulation that a miner's last year of service be in a union mine achieved the same end—it prevented older miners eligible for retirement from spending their last years in a nonunion mine. The trustees' actions showed a disregard for the fact that many of these miners had not only spent the requisite 20 years in union mines but had also, in many cases, been laid-off from their union jobs as a result of mechanization and a lack of seniority language in their contracts.

Miners and their families grew increasingly skeptical of the basis for the trustees' actions in altering eligibility rules. Rank-and-file concern was boosted considerably after the cutbacks in the 1960s which, for the first time, struck at the core of the union's membership. The stream of cutbacks issued by the trustees produced a burgeoning dissent movement within mining communities. During the 1960s, miners gained access to the Fund's financial records and began questioning the trustees' management of the union's finances. Moreover, miners began to go beyond scrutinizing individual decisions made by the trustees to questioning the process by which those decisions were reached. They increasingly viewed the decision-making structure that had propelled the union, under the firm hand of Lewis, to the fore of the labor movement as autocratic and out-of-touch with the needs of the rank-and-file.

Groups affected by the eligibility cuts mounted a series of legal challenges to win back their benefits. In 1965, by court order, the trustees reversed their 1953 decision requiring miners to accrue their 20 years of employment in union mines in the 30 years prior to retirement. Grassroots pressure was such that the following year Fund trustees headed off another court case and reinstated benefits to miners whose operators were behind in their royalty payments.[59] In general, however, the courts upheld the trustees' right to make decisions concerning the operation of the Fund. Plaintiffs eventually gained an advantage in 1968 when a federal appeals court ruled that decisions deemed "arbitrary and capricious" could be reviewed by the courts. As a result of that decision, in 1968 the courts ruled that the trustees' 1965 directive that a miner's last year be in a union mine in order to qualify for a pension was "unfair and unreasonable."[60]

The initial reductions in the size of the beneficiary pool stemming from the changes in eligibility rules and pension levels largely met the trustees' goal of reducing the Fund's expenditures. However, the policy changes also altered the composition of the beneficiary pool, although with less certain effects on the Fund's expenditures. The only policies that had easily discernable effects on the Fund's expenditures were those related to pensions and benefits for the disabled which removed some of the oldest and sickest people from the beneficiary pool. By contrast, the 1960 elimination of benefits of miners unemployed for more than a year, of self-employed miners, and of miners whose employers were behind in their royalty payments, accelerated the aging of the Fund's beneficiary pool by removing a large group of working miners from the pool.[61]

Furthermore, the reinstatement of beneficiaries when policies were reversed also had an ambiguous impact on the Fund's expenditures. Little is known about the sort of health care received in the interim by those who lost their Fund benefits. For example, it is possible that former beneficiaries simply went without health care, causing their medical conditions to develop to stages where they required costly, long-term attention when they returned to the Fund's care. Hence, the trustees' temporary removal of beneficiaries from the Fund's care may have adversely affected administrators' efforts to provide care in a cost-effective manner.

In addition to decreasing the size of the beneficiary pool, the Fund's other major bid to reduce costs was its sale of the Miners Memorial Hospitals. As the size of the beneficiary pool decreased, so too, had the proportion of Fund beneficiaries in the hospitals' patient base. As noted in chapter 5, the ratio of Fund beneficiaries was particularly low in the hospitals located in certain parts of eastern Kentucky (Whitesburg, McDowell, Hazard, Harlan, and Middlesboro) which had proportionately fewer unionized mines.[62] The rising proportion of non-beneficiaries in the hospitals was cause for concern as the Fund subsidized their care; Draper estimated that "the MMHA sustains an overall average loss of approximately 50 cents on every dollar in hospitalizing non-Fund patients."[63] Fund payments to the MMHA had risen steadily from $11.2 million in 1957 (18.9 percent of all medical expenditures in fiscal year 1957) to $17 million in 1962 (33.5 percent of all medical expenditures in fiscal year 1962).[64] In a period of declining income, the Fund's trustees concluded that they could no longer support an undertaking that so significantly drained the Fund's coffers.

In October 1962, the Fund's trustees announced their intention to sell the chain of hospitals. Anxious to keep the hospitals open in a region that lacked an adequate supply of comparable facilities, the board of the National Missions of the United Presbyterian Church established a nonprofit corporation, Appalachian Regional Hospitals, Inc. (ARHI), to buy the ten hospitals.[65] Using money provided by the church and funds obtained from the Commonwealth of Kentucky and President Kennedy's newly-created Area Redevelopment Administration, ARHI purchased the hospitals at Harlan, Hazard, McDowell, Middlesboro, and Whitesburg for $3.9 million in September 1963, and the hospitals at Man, Beckley, Pikeville, Williamson, and Wise for $4.1 million in June 1964. The total sale price of $8 million fell substantially short of the original $30 million cost of the chain's construction.

The trustees awaited a number of benefits from the sale of the hospitals. They expected the Fund's finances to improve not only from a cessation in the drain of funds to the MMHA, but also from the eventual transfer of funds from non interest-bearing mortgages into income-generating investments.[66] Moreover, the trustees took solace in the fact that the ARHI kept the hospitals functioning, thereby preserving both Fund beneficiaries' access to high quality care and the environment necessary to attract physicians to the coalfields. Many doctors originally recruited by the Fund to work in the hospitals stayed in the coalfields and continued to receive payments from the Fund. In addition, since the Fund continued to provide a large percentage of the hospitals' incomes, it retained a large role in maintaining standards in the hospitals.[67]

However, there were significant drawbacks to selling the hospital chain. First, the trustees' decision incurred considerable rank-and-file discontent. The construction of the Miners Memorial Hospitals had been a source of pride for miners and their families. In a very real sense the hospitals represented the sacrifices miners had made, particularly in the 1930s and 1940s, to build a union that raised living standards in communities whose fortunes were formerly dependent entirely on the operators who ran them. The trustees decision to sell the hospitals—and to sell them without consulting the rank-and-file—prompted wildcat strikes. Second, the sale of the hospitals cut short the Fund's experiment in operating its own hospitals. Administrators had been given only six years to attempt to operate the hospitals in a way that might have produced significant cost savings in the long term. Furthermore, the timing of the sale was particularly unfortunate since the inception of Medicare payments in the summer of 1966 may have afforded significant reductions in the cost of non-beneficiary care.

The Fund's strategy of trimming its beneficiary rolls and selling the Memorial Hospitals allowed it to survive the depression in the coal markets of the late 1950s and early 1960s, and to post healthy financial results for the remainder of the 1960s. In choosing this strategy, the Fund's trustees abandoned the vision of having the union provide cradle-to-grave support for miners and their families, whether working, disabled, unemployed, or retired. Yet the strategy was almost as remarkable for the approaches that it *did not* adopt as for the methods that it embraced. Curiously absent from the trustees' strategy were any proposals to increase the Fund's income or to alter its system of financing. These omissions were intentional and were a direct consequence of the compromise that Lewis had brokered in 1950.

Implications of the 1950 Compromise:
Expenditure Cuts Over Income Increases

The trustees' decision to eliminate the Fund's operating deficit by favoring expenditure reductions over income increases was an outgrowth of the alliance Lewis forged with large operators in 1950. Throughout his tenure as head of the union, Lewis remained convinced that the union was best served by bolstering the competitive position of operators capable of competing with alternative energy sources and nonunion mining operations. Intent on preserving the profitability of these large operators, Lewis refrained from proposing an increase in employer contributions—either through a raise in the royalty rate or a change in the financing mechanism—in order to remedy the Fund's financial difficulties.

Lewis's decisions concerning the Fund are better understood when viewed in the context of certain of his other decisions regarding the operation of the union and the management of its financial resources. Throughout the 1950s and 1960s, Lewis used union funds and staff to promote actively the interests of the large coal companies upon which he felt the future of the industry and, by extension, the union rested. Most notably, Lewis purchased controlling stock in the National Bank of Washington and placed all of the union's funds, including those of the Welfare and Retirement Fund, in the bank for use at his discretion. At Lewis's direction, the bank made loans to operators for mechanization, and to industrialist Cyrus Eaton for the purchase of nonunion mines in Kentucky with the stipulation that he recognize the union once he became their owner. Lewis also used the union's monies to purchase utility company stocks with the aim of pressuring them to buy union coal.[68] In addition, to ensure that production continued without disruption, Lewis refrained from calling work stoppages and clamped down on wildcat strikes.[69] Finally, Lewis placed Tony Boyle at the head of an "organizing" campaign designed to eliminate small nonunion mines concentrated in Kentucky and Tennessee. In essence, nonunion mines were given the choice of signing a UMWA contract and risking bankruptcy, or suffering physical destruction of their operations by "organizers."

What accounted for the abrupt change in Lewis's strategy from flexing union muscle by disrupting production to sponsoring illegal activities and manipulating high finance in a veiled alliance with large operators? As his biographers Melvyn Dubofsky and Warren Van Tine summarize,

> The diminished place of coal in the national economy, the changed nature of the industry itself, and the UMW's isolation from the larger

labor movement all served to transfer the union's source of power from its membership to its treasury. And, as the UMW's strength flowed solely from its purse, its values and structure changed. Lewis, at times unintentionally and unknowingly, acted to transform the UMW's primary concern from the welfare of its membership to the preservation of its treasury.[70]

In fact, preserving the treasury was not necessarily an end in itself. Rather, a strong treasury, Lewis felt, would best secure the union's future by allowing it to invest funds in areas that would protect the large operators. Thus, no "transformation" in priorities was necessary, although appearances certainly suggested otherwise.

Specifically, Lewis rejected three possible methods of increasing the Fund's income: increasing the royalty rate, transferring monies from the union's treasury, and altering the pay-as-you-go nature of the Fund. First, the suggestion that the royalty rate be increased from its 1952-level of 40 cents per ton was absent from contract negotiations until the 1970s. An increase in employer contributions while the coal market was in the recession of the 1950s would have had a significant impact on the competitiveness of large operators and might also have forced small operators to become nonunion or go out of business. However, the period between 1963 and 1972 witnessed renewed growth in coal demand—fueled primarily by consumption by electric utilities—and an end to the decline in coal's share of the energy market. Operators earned an average 3.5 percent return on investment in the period between 1963 and the first oil shock in 1972.[71]

Despite such indications that employers were in a position to increase their contributions to the Fund, the UMWA leadership allowed the royalty rate to continue to erode in real terms.[72] The union leadership's failure to demand an increase in the royalty rate was consistent with its continuing resistance to ask for concessions that would be unpopular with employers. Throughout the 1960s, miners noted the absence of proposals to increase the royalty rate for the Fund as a way of reversing the eligibility cuts that had been made in when the industry was flagging. Moreover, the timing of Fund's sale of its hospitals in 1963 and 1964 was particularly ironic given that the industry's concurrent recovery was not coupled with an increase in employer contributions to the Fund. The failure of the union to parlay the increase in its bargaining position into, among other things, an increase in the royalty rate would cause the rank-and-file to question openly the stewardship of the union.

Second, Lewis refused to tap into the UMWA's treasury for additional income for the Fund. By conservative estimates, in 1960 the union held

$17.7 million in investments and $56.7 million more in loans and notes receivable.[73] It is unlikely that Lewis was concerned with a possible conflict of interest in transferring monies between the union's treasury and the Fund; he had shown little concern for such possible conflicts in the much more dubious use of the treasury's monies to, for instance, make loans to operators. Instead, it appears that Lewis felt that the treasury should be used solely to shore up the industry which would then improve the Fund's position.

Third, Lewis declined to alter the pay-as-you-go nature of the Fund in order to stabilize its financial footing. As early as 1947, actuary reports advised the formation of a large trust fund to provide benefits for the lifetime of its beneficiaries. In order to build such a fund, the reports counseled the Fund to move away from its disbursement system in favor of an accumulation of reserves. The reports considered reserves to be "essential," especially given the unstable conditions in the coal industry.[74]

In fact, the Fund did build its reserves, but not with the intention of creating a trust fund for beneficiaries. The Fund did not even have a rule for minimum reserves, but attempted to increase reserves as much as possible.[75] The trustees' obsession with building reserves is evidenced by their actions in 1960, when the decline in reserves prompted them to cut eligibility. Put in perspective, the $99.8 million the Fund was left with in reserves was six times larger than its operating deficit. Moreover, it took the Fund only seven years to almost double these reserves (see Figure 16). While the practice of prioritizing the accumulation of reserves may seem unsound when examined solely in terms of the operations of the Fund, it was quite consistent with Lewis's other aims. Specifically, since the Fund's reserves were held in the union-controlled National Bank, they could be used to promote the union's other activities.

Finally, it is worth noting that Lewis avoided another avenue that might have improved the Fund's financial health, but at the expense of operators' competitiveness: increasing the attention paid to occupational health and safety. Injuries and illnesses produced in the mines created a tremendous burden on the Fund's expenditures, yet Lewis did not lobby for increased safety measures or dust control as these measures interfered with production. While the UMWA was the first union to establish an Office of Occupational Health, the leadership largely ignored its work until a grassroots movement formed around health and safety issues threatened rebellion.[76]

The control that Lewis exercised over the union put him squarely at the helm when the successful attainment of a solid contract in 1950 thrust the union into an industrial partnership with management. Lewis directed the union's affairs in a manner that precluded involvement in decision-making by others. There is no evidence that the Fund's other trustees, Josephine Roche and Henry Schmidt, ever challenged Lewis's decisions. Fund administrators appeared to be largely absent from discussions concerning eligibility cuts and the sale of the Memorial Hospitals. Finally, the Fund's beneficiaries were not consulted about policy changes even though, technically, Lewis was the rank-and-file's representative to the board.

How are we to assess Lewis's actions? Lewis had, after all, built a national reputation by championing the demands of coal miners. Yet his actions from 1950 until his death in 1969 appeared to have veered drastically from this course. Perhaps he was convinced that labor was in need of new strategies once the organizing push of the 1930s and 1940s had produced acceptable contracts. Perhaps he could think of no alternative to colluding with major producers as the reign of King Coal came to an end. Perhaps, as his biographers Dubofsky and Van Tine suggest, his vision was obscured by old age and declining health, increasing distance from the rank-and-file, and the desire to end his career as a labor leader revered not only by his membership, but by the leaders of government and industry.

The Fund's ambitious managed care program was affected by changes in the supply of and demand for health care brought about by opposition from organized medicine and changes in industry conditions. On the supply side, opposition from organized medicine diminished the ability of the Fund to recruit physicians to care for Fund beneficiaries, and to encourage them to adhere to the Fund's review practices and reimbursement policies. In addition, the trustees' decision to sell the Memorial Hospitals ended administrators' direct control of the supply of hospital services. On the demand side, changing industry conditions affected the needs of the Fund's beneficiaries through changes in the size and composition of the workforce, and changes in the hazards of production. In addition, the trustees' outright manipulation of eligibility rules for Fund services also altered the needs of the beneficiary pool.

It should be noted that while these trends are apparent in retrospect, it is unclear how evident they were to administrators during the Fund's first two decades of operation. Analyzing the ramifications of changes in production methods, industry conditions, and the Fund's finances would have come second to the formidable task of operating a comprehensive health plan of the Fund's magnitude. While the battle against the objections and obstacles posed by organized medicine took place on familiar terrain, the struggle to address changing industry conditions required a different kind of expertise.

While the failure of administrators to recognize these issues is evident with hindsight, it is important to realize the ease with which they could have been overlooked at the time that the administrators were busy creating, evaluating, and reforming the operation of the Fund. After all, questions of Fund finances and the fortunes of the mining population were left in the presumably capable hands of the man who negotiated the benefits in the first place: John L. Lewis. For his part, Lewis proved to be surprisingly incapable of understanding that the compromise he made in 1950 would have long-term consequences for the Fund's finances and the composition of the beneficiary pool. Central to the compromise, the Fund would bear the brunt of its effects.

CHAPTER SEVEN

The Transformation and Dismantling of the Fund

*T*he fate of the Fund in the 1970s was determined by the same forces that led to its creation in 1950: industry conditions and the relative bargaining positions of the operators and the union. The 1970s witnessed a resurgence in the demand for coal as a result of the OPEC price shocks and the ensuing energy crisis (see Figure 8). However, an increasing share of the demand for coal was supplied by nonunion, western strip mines with the result that the share of union coal fell from 74 percent of all coal production in 1968 to 50 percent of total production by 1977.[1] Competition from nonunion coal weakened the UMWA's bargaining position which, in turn, limited the demands the union could place on BCOA operators.

For their part, the BCOA operators had come a long way from the fractious days of the late 1940s. Two decades of cooperation aided by increasing concentration in the industry improved the internal cohesion of the BCOA. By contrast, the UMWA suffered the growing pains of moving from the autocratic style favored by Lewis to a more democratic mode of operation. The coalfields of the 1970s experienced rank-and-file rebellion that was aimed not only at their traditional opponents, the operators, but also at the reform-oriented leadership they had fought to install. The BCOA eventually used its unity to exploit the disarray within the UMWA and wrest control of the Fund away from the union.

The backlash against the leadership style of Lewis and his successor Tony Boyle also produced a new set of Fund trustees and directors. Lacking an appreciation of the Fund's historic commitment to managed care, this new administration gradually transformed the Fund into a more traditional third-party payer. Specifically, the AMOs were stripped of much of their ability to review and manage programs locally. The 1974 contract divided the Fund into four different trusts, separating the provision of pensions from health benefits and separating retired from working miners. This partitioning allowed the union leadership to engage in actions reminiscent of the 1960s, namely the privileging of a central over a marginal constituency of the beneficiary pool in order to address the growing cost of care.

The transformation of the Fund would be completed in 1977 when its leadership attempted to remedy financial troubles by implementing beneficiary copayments for the first time in the Fund's history. With the 1977 contract, the UMWA also relinquished control over the care of working and recently retired miners, thus ending the Fund's central place in the minds of working union members. What remained of the Fund was preserved only for older, retired miners.

Finally, a number of important issues must be examined before the transformation of the Fund in the 1970s is discussed. The introduction of Medicare in the late 1960s and the initiation of federal black lung disability compensation in the early 1970s targeted the Fund's oldest and sickest beneficiaries. While the importance of these programs deserves mention, they did not significantly reduce the Fund's formidable burden of providing medical care for the aged. Furthermore, changes in the industry's employment pool spawned by the increase in coal demand placed additional burdens on the Fund. The changing demographics of the workforce also provided operators with an opportunity to use the shape of the Fund as a wedge to divide the miners.

Caring for Older Beneficiaries

The late 1960s brought two changes which, on face value, should have brought financial relief to the Fund: Medicare and black lung legislation. While both programs targeted the growing number of aged and ailing members of the Fund's beneficiary pool, neither reduced expenditures to sustainable levels. First, as shown in Figure 14, the Medicare program appears to have reduced the Fund's outlays only in the first few years following its inception in mid-1966. By the early 1970s, a rapid escalation in the cost of medical care—no doubt spurred by the increase in demand fostered by the Medicare program itself—taxed the Fund's resources. It should be noted that the Fund continued to cover some of the costs of care for beneficiaries who were also Medicare recipients. Specifically, the Fund paid the co-insurance on Medicare policies and also for prescription drugs not covered by Medicare.

Second, as the result of a grassroots organizing campaign that brought national attention to the ravages of coal workers' pneumoconiosis, Congress passed the Federal Coal Mine Health and Safety Act of 1969. The act gave the Bureau of Mines greater authority to close unsafe mines, set tougher safety standards and mandated fines for violations, set maximum coal dust levels for the first time, and provided benefits to ailing miners and their families. While the contours of the black lung program were altered numerous times after its passage, it provided needed cash assistance for ailing miners and worked to reduce future incidence of the disease. However, the act did not include coverage of medical care with the result that the Fund continued to care for afflicted miners at an enormous cost. The relief, then, that the Fund could expect from a reduction in the incidence of black lung would only accrue in the long run.

While national policy initiatives did little to reduce the Fund's expenditures to sustainable levels, changes in the age profile of the Fund's beneficiary pool increased the drain on the Fund's monies. In the 1970s, employment in the industry increased as a result of both the resurgence in demand for coal and the decrease in productivity in underground mining.[2] As a result, the age distribution of the mining workforce shifted toward younger miners as the industry experienced a influx of approximately 118,000 new miners between 1969 and 1978 (see Figure 9), the vast majority of whom were young. Concurrently, 50,000 older miners retired in order to receive black lung disability benefits.[3] These two factors reversed the postwar trend and produced a younger mining workforce. For example, in eastern mines in 1969, more than half of the miners were older than 44 years and only one-fourth of miners were under 35 years old. By 1979 the proportions were reversed with only a fourth of the workforce over 44 years and half of the workforce under 35 years of age.[4]

Yet, while the employment pool became younger, the Fund's beneficiary pool continued to include older miners. The resulting age profile included a disproportionate number of the very young and the very old, two groups that place great demands on the health care system. Ironically, operators would exploit the difference in the age profiles between the pool of working miners and the pool of union members to help dismantle the Fund.

Administrative Changes

In the late 1960s, the operation of the Fund took a backseat to events that radically restructured the UMWA. The last two years of the decade witnessed a major mining disaster at Farmington, West Virginia, the death of John L. Lewis, a fierce campaign for the presidency of the UMWA that was later determined to be marred by fraud, the murder of insurgent candidate for UMWA presidency Joseph "Jock" Yablonsky and his family, and the rise of a grassroots movement that succeeded in gaining passage of federal black lung legislation. In addition, in 1969 a group of disabled miners who had been denied pensions were joined by a contingent of miners' widows and other Fund beneficiaries concerned about the future of their benefits in filing a class action suit alleging mismanagement of the Fund by the UMWA leadership. Three years later, the plaintiffs in *Blankenship v. Boyle* achieved victory in a decision that paved the way for a more democratic union leadership to emerge.[5]

The *Blankenship* decision condemned union leadership's practice of aiding the competitive position of BCOA operators at the expense of members' benefits. The revelation of these practices in court forced Tony Boyle and Josephine Roche to leave office, ending the era of close cooperation between union and industry leaders. *Blankenship* also led to an overhaul of the Fund's administration. In 1972 the UMWA's new president Arnold Miller appointed Harry Huge, the plaintiffs' attorney in *Blankenship*, to be the union's trustee on the Fund's board. Huge hired his friend Martin Danziger, a Justice department lawyer, to be the Fund's director.

Despite their prominence as attorneys, Huge and Danziger lacked experience in the management and administration of pensions and health care. Moreover, perhaps due to their desire to heed the lessons of *Blankenship*, Huge and Danziger promoted a management style that focused on procedure and downplayed the importance of the substantive programs upon which the Fund had built its reputation.[6] Daniel Marschall observed,

> With the union run as a dictatorship for fifty years, there was no opportunity for alternative leadership to grow from the rank and file and gain the kind of administrative experience necessary to govern a large, complex union effectively. Especially in a period when unions largely are not class-conscious organizations, and contain a variety of political tendencies, organizational expertise, political lobbying, and the ability to build coalitions among contending political forces are as important as sincere identification with membership interests. [The UMWA leadership] had never held high union office before. The reform officers confronted an immensely difficult task of both introducing democratic methods to union members who often had never known them, and developing a strong union that could face coal operators and the federal government as a unified force. It is not surprising that they succeeded only in part of that task.[7]

Fundamentally, the new leadership never fully understood the importance of the scope or the spirit of the Fund's programs as a key element in building cohesiveness in the union.

The first casualty of the new order was the role of the AMOs. Huge and Danziger instituted a drastic and sudden centralization and computerization of billing that disrupted the system of local administration that AMOs' staffs had carefully crafted. AMO administrators had spent years forging relations with providers, developing the medical care infrastructure of the coalfields, and carefully monitoring and reviewing providers' services and charges. Huge and Danziger subordinated the contributions of these skilled Fund veterans to their zeal to implement procedural reforms.[8]

The change in billing procedures slowed payments to a point where operations at clinics heavily dependent on Fund reimbursement were jeopardized. Moreover, local cost-containment efforts were hampered by the transfer of data to a central location. AMOs were forced to relax their pressure on local providers as 'reasonableness' in charges and service levels could no longer be checked as effectively. In addition, the new Fund leadership instituted cutbacks in administrative services that threatened administrators' ability to monitor the quality and costs of care. The Washington office trimmed field staff services, eliminated important outreach and referral services, and reduced technical assistance and aid to providers.[9] As a former health-service specialist with the Johnstown AMO summarized,

> Many costs and quality controls in the health program have been lost. Medical bills are paid late (if not lost); duplicate claims are paid; pension checks to retired miners are delayed; eligibility controls are often out of control. Virtually all experienced top-level staffers have been retired, fired, or have quit in disgust. In their place have come dozens of would-be technocrats who know nothing of labor, health or pension programs, or management. These technocrats don't stay long, however, and the incredible turnover fuels the problem. So much of the Funds' program has been gutted while it was 'modernized.' And direct health expenditures and administrative costs have risen dramatically.[10]

In just the two years between 1974 and 1976, administrative costs rose 90 percent and medical care costs rose 73 percent.[11] It appeared that the Fund's new directors had succeeded in replacing the autocratic governing style of the Fund's former trustees with a technocratic style that created its own problems. The administrative overhaul of the Fund in the early 1970s represented the first in a string of departures from the Fund's historic commitment to locally-administered efforts to increase the cost-effectiveness of care while preserving access to and quality of care. Ironically, the Fund's top administrators had begun stripping the Fund of the very programs and policies that would be implemented by its more conventional successors.

The 1974 Contract: Partitioning the Fund

As administrative changes stripped the Fund of much of its spirit, changes promulgated by the 1974 contract fundamentally altered the structure of the Fund.[12] The 1974 contract divided the Fund into four separate trusts.[13] Miners who retired before December 31, 1975, would receive health benefits from the 1950 Benefit Trust and pensions from the 1950 Pension Trust. Miners who retired after December 31, 1975, would receive health benefits from the 1974 Benefit Trust and pensions from the 1974 Pension Trust. While health benefits remained equal under the two Benefit Trusts, beneficiaries of the 1974 Pension Trust received higher pensions than retired miners covered by the 1950 Pension Trust.

In a further departure from parity across the beneficiary pool, the 1974 Trusts benefited from an improved financing mechanism. The tonnage royalty for the 1974 Trusts was supplemented by an employer contribution made on the basis of hours worked in classified (bargaining unit) jobs. The addition of the hour-based contribution enabled the Fund to recover some of the losses it had sustained from the decline in productivity that had begun in the late 1960s, and obviated the need for huge increases in the tonnage royalty rate. The effective royalty rate more than doubled as a consequence of the change in the financing mechanism.[14] Meanwhile, the 1950 Trusts continued to be financed strictly on a tonnage basis, although at higher tonnage royalty rates negotiated in both the 1971 and 1974 contracts.

In acceding to this restructuring, the UMWA leadership invoked the practice of sacrificing the benefits of a relatively more marginal segment of the beneficiary pool—in this case the older retired miners—in order to preserve and enhance the benefits of the central core of working miners. The UMWA leadership engaged in the same type of calculus that had been used by the previous regime to justify discriminatory actions like the eligibility cuts in the mid-1950s and early 1960s. For example, the leadership maintained that providing pensions at the 1974 levels for 80,000 retired miners would have necessitated a royalty increase that would have pushed marginal operations out of business. Moreover, UMWA leaders maintained that the prospect of shouldering the burden of a large group of retired miners was impeding organizing efforts of younger miners in Kentucky and in the west.[15]

In the years following the 1974 contract, financial problems plagued the weakest of the trusts, those designed to provide health benefits and pensions to miners who had retired before 1976. The tonnage royalty financing mechanism proved incapable, as it had in the past, of providing the income required to meet the formidable needs of the retired population. Expenditures were higher than had been expected by negotiators in 1974 due to an underestimate of the number of beneficiaries, an overestimate of projected coal production, higher than expected medical care inflation, and higher than expected administrative costs. In addition, the BCOA and UMWA leadership charged that a wave of wildcat strikes significantly reduced royalty payments.[16] Even a series of suspect reallocations of funds between the trusts did not manage to prevent the 1950 Trusts from careening toward bankruptcy by 1977.[17]

Faced with potential insolvency, the trustees instituted deductibles for the first time in the history of the Fund.[18] Beginning July 1, 1977, the trustees imposed a $250 deductible for hospital bills, and required beneficiaries to pay co-insurance of 40 percent for nonhospital care to a maximum of $500 per family. This policy change violated the Fund's former practice of eschewing financial incentives that had the potential of deterring beneficiaries from seeking specialist and hospital care when such care was recommended by a physician. However, the imposition of deductibles was reminiscent of previous policy changes that mandated reductions in expenditures instead of increases in income. In this sense, the policy change was consistent with practices that had been discredited in the reform wave of the late 1960s and early 1970s—practices that shifted the burden of increasing costs onto beneficiaries and preserved the competitiveness of the BCOA.

The trustees also eliminated retainer payments to providers and moved the Benefit Trusts toward reimbursement based solely on a fee-for-service basis. Danziger argued that the termination of retainer payments would eliminate cross-subsidization of non-beneficiaries and would remove the inequities that resulted when only a portion of the beneficiary pool had access to such care. In addition, Danziger noted that he could find no evidence to support the claim that retainer payments decreased costs through reducing hospitalization.[19]

Danziger's claims are not supported by a careful analysis of the Fund's record. First, while Fund administrators acknowledged the potential for cross-subsidization of non-beneficiaries through the use of retainer payments, there is no evidence to suggest that cross-subsidization was rampant or that it imposed an intolerable cost. As noted in chapter 4, Fund administrators were willing to underwrite a wide range of services supplied by retainer providers—especially in group practice settings—since these services increased the quality of care, and in many instances, were substitutes for more costly hospital care. In fact, if the clinics' range of services attracted non-beneficiaries, they served the additional purpose of widening the providers' patient base.

Second, Danziger's claim that the elimination of retainer payments reduced inequities in access to care across the beneficiary pool is specious. The Fund's use of retainer payments was intended largely to reduce excessive utilization and, therefore, would not have disadvantaged those beneficiaries who did not have access to retainer providers. There is no evidence that beneficiaries themselves perceived there to be any inequities if, in fact, they were even aware of the type of payment their providers received. Moreover, since retainer payments were instrumental in encouraging providers to establish practices in underdeveloped areas, the elimination of this stable source of income probably created inequities in access to care across the beneficiary pool. Providers in the coalfields that depended on the Fund as one of the few sources of guaranteed income available in these areas found that the termination of retainer payments disrupted their planning and threatened their financial viability. For instance, physician staffing at central Appalachian clinics dependent on Fund reimbursement fell 42 percent and nonphysician staffing there fell 25 percent in the first year after the removal of retainer payments.[20]

Third, as the evidence presented in chapter 4 attests, ample proof of the savings realized through the use of retainer payments was available. Retainer providers by and large supplied services at lower unit charges and engaged in less hospitalization than did their fee-for-service colleagues. In the end, the elimination of retainer payments appears have been based more on the exigencies of billing than on cost and equity arguments. Retainer payments were difficult to reconcile with the individual billing required to charge copayments.[21]

With the implementation of deductibles and co-insurance and the elimination of prepayment in favor of fee-for-service reimbursement, the Benefit Trusts began to resemble more traditional third-party insurers than their predecessor, the Fund. While conflicting with the practices the Fund was best known for, these policy changes were consistent with the new administration's centralization of billing and constriction of the role of the AMOs. The transformation of the Fund was nearly complete as the managed care initiatives that previous Fund administrators had crafted to achieve their objectives were either eliminated entirely or rendered impotent.

The 1977 Contract: Dismantling the Fund

By 1977, the bargaining positions of the UMWA and the BCOA were diametrically opposed to those that had existed during the collective bargaining process that had produced the Fund in the late 1940s. The BCOA was now unified as a result of three decades of joint action and of the increasing concentration of the industry. The process of concentration that had begun with the help of Lewis had continued into the 1970s as oil companies began buying coal companies. In the 1970s, the 5 percent of all mines that produced more than 500,000 tons of coal accounted for half of all production, while the 80 percent of mines that produced less than 100,000 tons produced only 20 percent of all coal.[22]

By contrast, the UMWA was in disarray. The union's leadership was weak and badly affected by anti-miner media.[23] The strikes that disrupted the industry were not the orchestrated protests that had occurred under John L. Lewis but, instead, wildcat strikes that expressed rising rank-and-file discontent with the union leadership. The democratization movement within the UMWA that had succeeded in removing a corrupt and autocratic leadership had installed a new leadership that, perversely, seemed just as distant from the membership.

In addition, the market for coal in the late 1970s was significantly different from that which had existed three decades earlier. Operators and utilities held large stockpiles that allowed them to withstand long strikes, and the competition provided by alternative fuels and nonunion coal greatly circumscribed the UMWA's ability to disrupt the energy market. Ironically, the inability of the UMWA to threaten seriously the nation's energy supply was exposed when a federal judge refused to extend a temporary Taft-Hartley back-to-work order in 1978 due to the lack of a national energy crisis.[24] Thus, even the impact of state intervention was different when President Jimmy Carter's tepid intercession in collective bargaining was compared to President Truman's seizure of the mines in the late 1940s.

Where the power of the UMWA's position and John L. Lewis's vision resulted in the creation of the Fund, the weakness of the union and its leadership's ineptitude resulted in the demise of the Fund's successors. As part of the 1977 contract, operators were given the responsibility of providing health care and pension benefits for working miners and miners who retired after 1975. Most employers contracted conventional third-party insurers to provide this coverage. The UMWA continued to cover the health and pension benefits primarily of those retired miners eligible for care under the

1950 Trusts. In addition, the 1974 Trusts continued to care for the relatively small group of miners whose last signatory employers were out of business and either qualified for pensions, were disabled after December 5, 1974, or had been laid-off.[25]

In addition, the deductibles that had been imposed earlier in the year as a temporary measure were codified in the contract. The deductibles were reduced somewhat so that working miners were now responsible for $200 of the costs of physician care and medication per year and retired miners were responsible for $100 of these costs per year. The dismantling of the Fund was now all but complete. Beneficiaries either were cared for by third-party insurers or received a similar type of coverage under the 1950 Trusts.

The BCOA enjoyed a number of advantages from assuming the care of working miners and recent retirees. First, eager to escape from the expensive burden imposed by the 1974 contract, operators expected to reduce the cost of care by curtailing benefits and introducing copayments. The deductibles alone were projected to save the BCOA $70 to $75 million per year.[26] Concurrently, the BCOA left the formidable problem of caring for older retirees to the union. Second, the BCOA was now in a position to realize the returns to worker loyalty that resulted from providing benefits more directly. The BCOA had agreed to give the union the control of the Fund in 1950 in return for the labor stability John L. Lewis could provide. With the UMWA leadership unable to control the rank-and-file, there was no reason for the BCOA to forgo the returns to worker loyalty that the provision of benefits could supply. Without a strong union leadership, the BCOA was in a position to assume greater control of the workforce by, among other things, providing working miners and recent retirees with pensions and health benefits.

The reasons for the UMWA's willingness to give up the Fund are less discernable and await more thorough historical analysis. At a minimum, the leadership's abdication of the 1974 Trusts can be viewed as a logical conclusion to its transformation of the Fund in the 1970s. The UMWA leadership's commitment to the Fund had waned once administrators left and took with them a coherent vision of the Fund's role in providing health care. Throughout the 1970s, the Fund ceased to be an effective tool of either the leadership to promote greater cohesion within the union, or of administrators to promote a progressive health policy agenda. The changes to the spirit and structure of the Fund combined with the declining prominence of the UMWA made the Fund increasingly untenable. Finally, in some sense it was unsurprising that as the UMWA withdrew from the forefront of labor movement, it also abandoned its attempt to marshal a pathbreaking health plan.

The Legacy of the Fund

The Fund deserves a significant place in history for its contribution to the development of modern health systems and for its pivotal role in shaping labor relations in the coal industry. As an unprecedented experiment in health care policy, Fund administrators designed and implemented managed care initiatives that were well ahead of their time. In addition, the Fund greatly increased beneficiaries' access to care of a commendable quality. In a relatively short period of time, the Fund replaced the inadequate company doctor system with a plan that was truly enviable. Miners and their families were given access to the country's foremost rehabilitation centers, best doctors, and a state-of-the-art chain of hospitals built right in the heart of Appalachia.

The Fund was less successful in maximizing the cost-effectiveness of care. In part, the Fund's cost of care was high for reasons beyond its control: the underdevelopment of the health care infrastructure in the coalfields and the formidable needs of the Fund's beneficiaries. In addition, the Fund's lack of coverage for primary care also played a role in curtailing its ability to decrease unnecessary utilization. However, the Fund's efforts still provide instructive alternative models of medical care delivery, particularly for providers caring for populations with demanding health needs living without access to quality care. Most notably, the Fund's use of physician panels and prepayment plans combined cost savings with high quality care. In fact, the contribution of these programs is evidenced by the impact of their withdrawal in the 1970s. The curtailment of AMO activity and the removal of retainer payments caused severe disruption in the provision of care in the areas most dependent on Fund direction and payments.

The fortunes of the Fund are also important as they present a reflection of the changing tide of labor relations within the coal industry. The Fund first was placed on the bargaining table when the price and wage freezes of World War II eliminated other concessions that would have ensured stable production during a period of high demand for coal. John L. Lewis was able to secure the Fund in 1950 as a result of the union's ability to disrupt the energy market and its ability to garner the support of the government and the conscience of the public. However, the procurement of the Fund came with the recognition that the UMWA would not enjoy either of these capabilities indefinitely. The growing competition from alternative fuels and small nonunion mines required Lewis to accept the Fund on the condition that the union agree to further mechanization of the mines.

The Fund, then, was central to industry peace during the 1950s and 1960s. Operators allowed Lewis to control the Fund and reap the returns to loyalty that resulted from its operation. Lewis, in exchange, operated the Fund without demanding additional employer contributions beyond the 40 cent royalty negotiated in 1950. In addition, Lewis sought to maximize the returns to beneficiary loyalty by promoting the Fund in a high-profile manner, emphasizing specialist and hospital care at the expense of primary physician care. The inability of the union leadership to reconcile the provision of such care with the demands of industrial partnership was demonstrated by the eligibility cuts scattered throughout the first two decades of the Fund's operation.

The events of the 1970s ended both the UMWA leadership's cooperation with the BCOA and the Fund's promotion of innovative, high-profile initiatives. The UMWA's ability to benefit from the rebound in the coal market was dampened by the continued competition from alternative fuels and the growing competition from large nonunion surface mining operations. The industrial partnership crafted by Lewis and honored by Boyle contained the seeds of its own demise as the direction of the union under this arrangement ultimately was determined to be unacceptable to the rank-and-file. The new leadership, however, proved incapable of preserving the Fund in the face of new conditions in the industry. Ironically, the reform leadership elected to depose autocratic rule resorted to many of the same tactics that the movement that had brought it to power had worked to uncover and discredit.

The dismantling of the Fund in 1977 did not, however, remove the union's provision of health benefits from the center of labor relations in the coalfields. The 1989 Pittston strike demonstrated the continued potency of retiree health care as a collective bargaining issue. Miners received national attention when they stopped work in protest of the Pittston Coal Company's refusal to make contributions to the Benefit Trusts and its termination of retiree health benefits. The resolve of the mining community in this long, bitter, and ultimately victorious strike displayed the importance of health benefits to miners and their families.

Finally, the events of the late 1940s unexpectedly resurfaced in Congress and the federal courts in 1992. A combination of events had pushed both Benefit Trusts into enormous operating deficits that the courts ruled could not be rectified by a proposed suspension of benefits. Congress eventually passed a bill, over the vociferous objections of western senators, that levied a tax on both union and nonunion coal mining operations in order to provide funds for the Benefit Trusts. The courts ruled that the federal government was within its rights to levy this tax even on nonunion operations because of its role in the establishment of the Fund in the late 1940s. Thus the extraordinary events that had produced the Krug-Lewis Agreement in 1947 were invoked 45 years later to secure the benefits of retired miners through an unusual tax scheme that spread the costs of mining coal across the entire industry.

In retrospect, many of the Fund's flaws and its ultimate incompatibility with other union objectives are apparent. However, throughout the 1940s, 1950s, and 1960s, the UMWA was the standard-bearer for an unprecedented new manner of providing health care—employer-financed and union-controlled—that still stands without equal. The UMWA faced a daunting task in providing health care to a neglected group of workers and their families in a vastly underdeveloped setting. Yet Fund administrators boldly embraced John L. Lewis's challenge to provide beneficiaries with the best care possible. They used previously untried ideas to construct a system of care that focused on access and quality without losing sight of costs. In doing so, the Fund developed a record that has earned it a distinctive place in both the evolution of health systems as well as in the history of the labor movement in the United States.

Data Sources

A comprehensive look at the Fund's performance is made possible by the wealth of data available in the Fund's Archives at the West Virginia and Regional History Collection in the West Virginia University Library. The Fund Archives contain a variety of internal reports, memoranda, and letters produced by Fund administrators from the inception of the Fund until 1974. This extraordinary collection provides fertile ground for researchers to examine questions beyond those addressed in this study.

Most of the data analyzed in this study comes from reports prepared by the Fund's Office of Research and Statistics (Series V). General data on beneficiaries' use of medical services come primarily from annual "Statistical Reports" prepared by the office. Annual reports on the proportion of hospital services used by Fund beneficiaries in relation to total hospital services provided in each Area Medical Office were also used to calculate beneficiary use of hospital services relative to that of local populations. The experience of the retainer payment program was analyzed using annual and monthly data on services and treatment included in the office's "Statistical Report Series—Summary of Retainers" reports.

The Office of Research and Statistics also issued annual reports on the experience of each of the Memorial Hospitals and for the chain as a whole. In addition, the archives also include documents and reports prepared by the staff of the MMHA itself (Series IV). This series includes correspondence concerning efforts to increase utilization of the Memorial Hospitals as well as the budgets for the hospitals.

Financial data comes primarily from the Fund's *Annual Reports* as well as from the Office of Research and Statistics, "Statistical Abstract" series. Finally, correspondence and reports on a variety of other issues can be found in the papers of the Office of the Executive Medical Officer (Series III).

Most notably, information on the Medical Management programs of the 1960s as well as information on the operation of the Fund in individual areas ("Information Reports") is included in correspondence between the AMOs and the Fund's national office.

In addition, this study makes use of documents available in the papers of Lorin Edgar Kerr, the UMWA's director of occupational health, and of Robert Kaplan, the Fund's research director. Both of these collections are housed at the Manuscripts and Archives Collection at Yale University.

Notes

CHAPTER ONE

1. In other industrializing nations, workers were more likely to receive health care from the state. European models of "social medicine" proffered a more comprehensive view of health, incorporating the impact of social factors in addition to biological factors in the study of the causes of illness. By integrating preventive medicine with the study of disease, the European model was better suited to public intervention and social insurance programs. By contrast, the American model of medical care provision evolved from "scientific" or laboratory-based science. The professionalization of medical care in the United States consequently spawned specialized fields of health care, separating, for instance, public health from physician care. The prevailing individualist ideology in the United States, moreover, relegated social medicine to care addressing problems generated by industry, urbanization, and immigration. Lily Hoffman, *The Politics of Knowledge: Activist Movements in Medicine and Planning* (Albany: State University of New York Press, 1989), 15.

2. Raymond Munts, *Bargaining for Health: Labor Unions, Health Insurance, and Medical Care* (Madison: University of Wisconsin Press, 1967), 6; and James B. Kennedy, "Beneficiary Features of American Trade Unions" (Ph.D. diss., Johns Hopkins University, 1907), 11–15. This perspective would also compel the American Federation of Labor (AFL), and particularly its president Samuel Gompers, to oppose state attempts to strip labor of an important source of labor cohesion through the provision of health benefits. Paul Starr, *The Social Transformation of American Medicine* (New York: Basic Books, 1982), 251; and Alan Derickson, "Health Security for All? Social Unionism and Universal Health Insurance, 1935–1958," *Journal of American History* 80 (March 1994): 1337. The argument that unions were more likely to ensure worker well-being was particularly persuasive in an era when the state did not enjoy a reputation as friend and protector of labor.

3. Jerome Schwartz, "Early History of Prepaid Medical Care Plans," *Bulletin of the History of Medicine* 39 (September–October 1965): 453.

4. Alan Derickson, *Workers' Health, Workers' Democracy: The Western Miners' Struggle, 1891–1925* (Ithaca: Cornell University Press, 1988).

5. Schwartz, 454.

6. Anna Kalet, "Voluntary Health Insurance in New York City," *American Labor Legislation Review* 6 (June 1916): 142–54.

7. Lee Janis and Milton I. Roemer, "Medical Care Plans for Industrial Workers and Their Relationship to Public Health Programs," *American Journal of Public Health* 38 (September 1948): 1246–47.

8. H. David Banta and Samuel J. Bosch, "Organized Labor and the Prepaid Group Practice Movement," *Archives of Environmental Health* 29 (July 1974): 44.

9. Munts, 30.

10. Interestingly, these conditions prompted the development of the nation's first health maintenance organization, Kaiser-Permanente. In the 1930s, industrial magnate Henry Kaiser contracted physicians to care for construction workers laboring in the Arizona desert. The success of this comprehensive plan lead to its expansion into a chain of providers available to all employee groups.

11. Roy Lubove, "Workmen's Compensation and the Prerogatives of Voluntarism," *Labor History* 8 (Fall 1967): 264.

12. Ibid., 271–72.

13. Peter Temin, "An Economic History of American Hospitals," in (ed.) H. E. Frech, *Health Care in America.* (San Francisco: Pacific Research Institute for Public Policy, 1988), 84.

14. Starr, 201.

15. Herman M. Somers and Anne R. Somers, *Doctors, Patients, and Health Insurance: The Organization and Financing of Medical Care* (Washington, D.C.: The Brookings Institution, 1961), 230.

16. Stuart D. Brandes, *American Welfare Capitalism* (Chicago: University of Chicago Press, 1976), 97.

17. Somers and Somers, 230.

18. Starr, 200–203.

19. Brandes, 99.

20. Most of the associations were between 10 and 14 years old and only 2 percent were more than 50 years old. U.S. Treasury Department, "A Survey of the Work of Employees' Mutual Benefit Associations," by Dean K. Brundage, *Public Health Reports* 46 (4 September 1931): 2102–13.

21. Ibid., 2112.

22. Ibid., 2119.

23. Ibid., 2112–13, 2119.

24. Schwartz, 461.

25. The Wagner Act (1935) established guidelines for contract negotiations. Besides wages and hours, the act vaguely referred to "other conditions of employment" as acceptable bargaining issues.

26. The first collectively bargained health plans most commonly provided cash benefits in case of sickness and disability. Coverage for hospitalization and surgical costs was somewhat less common and coverage for physician care was rare. Florence Peterson, Everett Kassalow, and Jean Nelson, "Health Benefit Programs Established Through Collective Bargaining," *Monthly Labor Review* 61 (August 1945): 191–209. Of the workers receiving coverage in 1948, roughly 11 percent received pension benefits only, 45 percent received health benefits only, and the remaining 44 percent received both health and pension benefits. U.S. Congress, Senate, Report of the Joint Committee on Labor-Management Relations, 80th Cong., 2d sess., 1948, 3–4.

27. The provision of medical care in the Armed Forces during World War II also gave physicians and the public a sense of the returns to greater organization of medical care. Servicemen and servicewomen received comprehensive care, some for the first time, through a centrally organized plan. Physicians employed by the armed forces and policymakers both noted that salaried medicine and group practice appeared to increase the quality and decrease the cost of care. Hoffman, 38.

28. Employer-financed plans were more prevalent among AFL unions than among CIO unions. Evan Keith Rowe, "Employee-Benefit Plans Under Collective Bargaining, Mid-1950," *Monthly Labor Review* 72 (February 1951): 159–61.

29. U.S. Department of Health, Education, and Welfare, Public Health Service, Division of Community Health Services, "Medical Care Financing and Utilization," *Health Economics Series* no. 1. (Washington, D.C.: GPO, 1962): Table 84, 96.

30. Ibid., Tables 84 and 85, 96–97; and Alfred M. Skolnik, "Employee-Benefit Plans: Developments, 1954–63," *Social Security Bulletin* 28 (April 1965): Table 2, 7.

31. A small number of unions attempted to mirror health-insurers by paying indemnity benefits based on fee schedules. John Simons, "The Union Approach to Health and Welfare," *Industrial Relations* 4 (May 1965): 63.

32. Comprehensive medical care was available at Union Health Service, Inc. in Chicago and the Labor Health Institute in St. Louis. American Medical Association, Council on Medical Service, "Union Health Centers, 1958 Survey," *Journal of the American Medical Association* 168 (1 November 1958): 1234–38.

CHAPTER TWO

1. U.S. Coal Mines Administration, *A Medical Survey of the Bituminous-Coal Industry* (Washington, D.C.: GPO, 1947), 120.

2. Leslie Falk, "Coal Miners' Prepaid Medical Care in the United States—and Some British Relationships, 1792–1964," *Medical Care* 4 (January 1966): 39.

3. Bureau of Cooperative Medicine, *Medical Care in Selected Areas of the Appalachian Bituminous Coal Fields* (New York: Bureau of Cooperative Medicine, 1939), 5. The UMWA asked the bureau to research the state of medical care in the coal fields. The study was funded by the Good Will Fund of Boston and the Twentieth Century Fund of New York. The bureau interviewed 787 miners and miners' wives, 75 doctors, and visited 38 hospitals in southern West Virginia and adjacent areas of Virginia, Kentucky, and Tennessee.

4. Ibid., 10.

5. U.S. Coal Mines Administration, 123.

6. Ibid., 124.

7. "Baker Finds Medical Care Inadequate," *United Mine Workers Journal*, 1 April 1946, 9. E. L. Baker, an UMWA negotiating committee member researching medical conditions in the coalfields in 1946, noted, "These big red pills . . . are generally known throughout the Southern mining industry as 'doorknobs' because they are so big you can hardly swallow them." Robert Kaplan, "The United Mine Workers' Welfare and Retirement Fund: Its Background and History," Ms, Robert Kaplan papers, Manuscripts and Archives, Yale University, New Haven, 34.

8. Most operators carried workers' compensation insurance which based the premiums on experience rating. Since premiums were based on the compensation paid out in the previous year, operators had an incentive to minimize the amount that they paid out in compensation claims. Companies minimized their liabilities by preventing company doctors or hospitals heavily used by miners from sending bills for medical care to the compensation fund (thus leaving the miner to underwrite the cost of care), or by encouraging providers to send bills which covered only a fraction of the cost of care. Bureau of Cooperative Medicine, 29–30. Moreover, operators pressed doctors to return injured miners to work as soon as possible in order to reduce the indemnity outlay. Even when medical care was received, obtaining cash benefits was difficult. Companies often argued that cases were not compensable by claiming that diagnoses were attributable to natural

causes, unrelated diseases or unsafe practices. In the case of death, the operators sometimes argued that death in a mining accident was the result of natural causes or even suicide. Kaplan, 28. Company doctors often had little choice in acceding to operators' demands. For instance, an operator fired a doctor who stated that a miner's death was due to a work-related injury rather than to natural causes as the company maintained. Bureau of Cooperative Medicine, 8.

9. David Alan Corbin, *Life, Work, and Rebellion in the Coal Fields* (Urbana: University of Illinois Press, 1981), 135, and Bureau of Cooperative Medicine, 9.

10. John L. Lewis, Statement before Senate Labor and Public Welfare Committee, 7 March 1947, reprinted in *United Mine Workers Journal* 58 (15 March 1947): 16.

11. Marjorie Taubenhaus and Roy Penchansky, "The Medical Care Program of the United Mine Workers Welfare and Retirement Fund," in *Health Services Administration: Policy Cases and the Case Method,* ed. Roy Penchansky (Cambridge: Harvard University Press, 1968), 157.

12. Kaplan, 29.

13. Bureau of Cooperative Medicine, 7.

14. U.S. Congress, Senate, Subcommittee of the Committee on Education and Labor, *A Resolution to Investigate Violations of the Right of Free Speech and Assembly and Interference with the Right of Labor to Organize and Bargain Collectively,* 75th Cong., 1st sess., 30 April, 3–5 May 1937, Harlan County: 4517.

15. "Paul K. Reed Tells Shocking Story of Disappearance of Insurance Rebates," *United Mine Workers Journal,* 1 April 1946: 6.

16. Bureau of Cooperative Medicine, 7.

17. "Vales Reveals How Coal Operators, Medical Associations Dominate Kentucky Doctor Setup," *United Mine Workers Journal,* 15 August 1947: 1.

18. Congress, Senate, Subcommittee of the Committee on Education and Labor, 4517.

19. Falk, 39.

20. This strike by 500 miners at the Paint Creek Collieries came only two months after the conclusion of the famous Paint Creek–Cabin Creek strike. Operators had originally agreed to remove the doctor in question at the conclusion of the first strike. Miners struck a second time when the operators reneged on that part of the agreement. Corbin, 135.

21. Bureau of Cooperative Medicine, 18–19, 54.

22. Donald Miller and Richard E. Sharpless, *The Kingdom of Coal: Work, Enterprise, and Ethnic Communities in the Mine Fields* (Philadelphia: University of Pennsylvania Press, 1985), 113.

23. Dorothy Schwieder, Joseph Hraba, and Elmer Schwieder, *Buxton: Work and Racial Equality in a Coal Mining Community* (Ames: Iowa State University Press, 1987), 78–79.

24. The President's Commission on Coal, *The American Coal Miner* (Washington, D.C.: GPO, 1980), 77.

25. Bureau of Cooperative Medicine, 22–25.

26. "'Pluck Me' Profit System Follows Dead Miner Right into Undertaking Parlor," *United Mine Workers Journal,* 1 April 1946: 7.

27. Bureau of Cooperative Medicine, 18.

28. Kaplan, 35.

29. Emphasis in the original. Bureau of Cooperative Medicine, 4.

30. J. Davitt McAteer, *Coal Mine Health and Safety* (New York: Praeger Publishers, 1970), 29.

31. Starr, 335.

32. The return on investment is the after tax return on total assets. Peter Navarro, "Union Bargaining Power in the Coal Industry, 1945–1981," *Industrial and Labor Relations Review* 36 (January 1983): 228.

33. The establishment of a health plan had been included in UMWA convention platforms since 1938 not so much as a concrete bargaining demand but rather as a protest of Congress's opposition to national health insurance. Lewis had raised concerns over health plans in the coalfields only once before the 1945 negotiations during the negotiations in 1941. At that time, however, his demands were restricted to allowing miners to participate in the management of the programs financed by their check-off deductions. Curtis Seltzer, *Fire in the Hole: Miners and Managers in the American Coal Industry* (Lexington: The University of Kentucky, 1985), 58. The bargaining process in the coal industry was highly centralized until the 1970s. The UMWA was virtually the only union that represented miners and contracts were negotiated on an industry-wide basis. During the period discussed in this chapter, UMWA membership is generally estimated to have exceeded 90 percent of the mining workforce. Moreover, within the union itself, control was concentrated centrally. By combining his force of personality with the union's constitutional provisions, John L. Lewis wielded enormous authority.

34. Justin McCarthy, "A Brief History of the UMWA," *United Mine Workers Journal,* 15 August 1957: 18.

35. Peterson, Kassalow, and Nelson, 191–209.

36. Melvyn Dubofsky and Warren Van Tine, *John L. Lewis* (New York: Quadrangle/ The New York Times Book Co., 1977), 459.

37. Seltzer, 58.

38. Miners were already among the highest paid industrial workers. The contracts negotiated during the late 1940s included only relatively modest wage increases, largely to keep pace with inflation. Navarro, 219.

39. "Affidavits Reveal the Tragic Story of Inadequate Compensation for Miners," *United Mine Workers Journal,* 15 April 1946: 7, 17; "'It's About Time We Got a Break,' says Injured Miner Who Can't Get Medical Care," *United Mine Workers Journal,* 15 May 1946: 9.

40. "It's about Time," 9.

41. Dubofsky and Van Tine, 460–61.

42. During his tenure as the government's representative in control of the mines, Krug did pick up the pace of mine safety inspections, but not enough to satisfy mine safety proponents.

43. Victims of mining disasters merit a prominent place in mining culture. The Fund's first payments went to 99 families affected by the Centralia disaster in the form of $1,000 death benefit checks.

44. There were roughly 7,000 mines and 400,000 miners in the industry at the time. Thus the report surveyed approximately 4 percent of all mines and 18 percent of all miners.

45. U.S. Coal Mines Administration, 116, 138.

46. Small mines rarely had a beneficiary pool of a size sufficient to attract physicians or hospitals. Moreover, most small mines were marginal producers that employed the most destitute of workers. These workers were among the least likely to be able to afford even a modest check-off for medical services.

47. U.S. Coal Mines Administration, 132.

48. Ibid., 156.

49. Ibid., 131.

50. Ibid., 154.

51. Ibid., 127.

52. Ibid.

53. Ibid., 191.

54. Ibid., 164.

55. Dubofsky and Van Tine, 472–73.

56. The Krug-Lewis Accord originally had mandated separate plans for the pension and health components of the Fund. These plans were merged under the 1947 agreement. Also, the separate health plan was originally intended to be managed by the union alone. However, the Taft-Hartley Act (passed just prior to the 1947 agreement) prevented unions from having sole control of benefit plans and mandated that control be shared equally with management.

57. Joseph Finley describes Van Horn as a "dour, elderly operator . . . a man as determined and unyielding as John L. Lewis . . . a man whose mere presence and attitude could frustrate the Fund." Joseph E. Finley, *The Corrupt Kingdom: The Rise and Fall of the United Mine Workers* (New York: Simon and Schuster, 1972), 180. The operators also had plans to litigate under the Taft-Hartley Act and lobby for congressional regulation of benefit plans in order to stop the operation of the Fund. Dubofsky and Van Tine, 476–77.

58. Murray was president of the Metropolitan Engineering Co. of Brooklyn, and a director of both the Chrysler Corporation and the Bank of New York. He had also acted as trustee of the Interborough Transit Company of New York and was credited with directing its successful reorganization during a period of financial difficulty. "Bituminous Welfare and Retirement Fund Set in Motion After Ten Months' Delay," *United Mine Workers Journal,* 15 May 1946: 9.

59. The three trustees argued primarily over the scope of the pension benefits that the Fund would provide. Murray and Lewis were closer to agreement than Van Horn. Murray and Lewis's proposals suggested different amounts of funding for the pensions but both made all union miners eligible for pensions. Van Horn not only rejected the levels of funding proposed, but also argued that eligibility be restricted to miners who retired from firms actually under contract. Dubofsky and Van Tine, 477.

60. Ibid., 483.

61. By the mid-1950s, the TVA would become the single largest consumer of coal in the United States. Seltzer, 73.

62. Van Horn disagreed with this decision and resigned. His motives were unclear but it is possible that he wanted to run the Fund into the ground by continuing the payments.

63. Captive mines are mines that are owned by large industrial producers like those in the steel industry. As such they are part of vertically integrated firms.

64. Interestingly, Truman had received reports from the Bureau of Mines that revealed that the nation's energy supply was not in fact facing imminent danger. The same forces that had worked to weaken operators' profits—competition from alternative fuels, reductions in exports, and undercutting by small mines—had worked to weaken the impact of the UMWA's disruption.

65. Seltzer maintains that both the operators and the union feared government intervention could go so far as to follow Europe's lead and nationalize the coal industry. These fears were not unfounded as the state of Virginia experimented with setting up local fuel

commissions to do everything from mining to selling and distributing coal during the wave of strikes in late 1949 and early 1950. Seltzer, 61.

66. Long-term contracts would account for about 80 percent of coal firms' contracts with utilities by the mid-1970s. Seltzer, 84, n. 71.

67. The UAW-General Motors contract that also was negotiated in 1950 incorporated many of these same features. The contract duration was lengthened to an unprecedented five years to allow GM to plan labor costs during a period of high growth. In addition, auto workers' compensation was linked directly to the firm's productivity through a wage escalator clause and an annual productivity increase. In return, the UAW received a union shop. As in the coal industry, the contract made it worthwhile for both management and labor to stabilize labor relations in the industry in an attempt to smooth production flows in a period of booming demand for automobiles. Nelson Lichtenstein, *Labor's War at Home: The CIO in World War II* (Cambridge: Cambridge University Press, 1982), 241.

68. Hubert Marshall, "Annual Report for 1954," memo to Warren Draper, 30 June 1955, 3, Fund Archives.

69. Kaplan, 4.

70. There were at least two precedents for the tonnage royalty payment system in the U.S. coal industry. The 1928 wage agreement between the coal operators in Wyoming and 5,000 miners represented by District 22 included an agreement by the operators to pay a half of a cent for each ton of coal mined into a fund that would cover medical care for mining injuries. Falk, 40. The Lehigh Coal and Navigation Company, an anthracite coal operator, financed its benefit fund through a combination of a tonnage royalty contribution and a tax of between .25 percent and .50 percent on the earnings of miners. In the period from 1884 to 1901, slightly more than half of the total contributions came from the company with the remainder from the workers. Ray Ginger, "Company-Sponsored Welfare Plans in the Anthracite Industry Before 1900," *Bulletin of the Business Historical Society* 27 (June 1953): 114–15.

71. In the spring of 1946, a report in the *United Mine Workers Journal* noted that payroll taxes were levied on Belgian producers to provide benefits for their workers. However, the report also suggested that tonnage royalties were a more common form of contribution to welfare funds given their use in Great Britain, British India, the Netherlands, Spain, and New Zealand. "Health and Welfare Funds for Miners are Common Throughout the Civilized World," *United Mine Workers Journal*, 1 June 1947: 18. Basing the financing mechanism on the amount of coal production turned out to be superior to basing it on the number of miners. The number of miners decreased steadily after 1953 until the 1970s. While union coal production also decreased from 1957 to 1961, it declined at a slower rate. Coal production then increased steadily after 1961.

72. The increases were necessary to allow the Fund to provide comprehensive benefits based on revisions to the budget projections once the Fund began operations. The royalty rate subsequently remained at the 1952 level until 1971 (see chapter 6).

73. Office of Technology Assessment, *The Direct Use of Coal* (Washington, D.C.: GPO, 1979), 133. Large operators and the union would combine efforts to drive out small mines again in the late 1950s when they lobbied together for stricter mine safety laws which were prohibitively expensive for smaller mines. It should be noted, however, that not all small mines were nonunion. Since these strategies did not discriminate, many small union mines were forced out of business.

74. John Peter David, "Earnings, Health, Safety, and Welfare of the Bituminous Coal Miners Since the Encouragement of Mechanization by the UMW of A," (Ph.D. diss., University of West Virginia, 1972), 231.

75. McCarthy, 14.

76. D. J. Kindel, "High Lights of the Medical and Health Program of the Consolidation Coal Company, Inc., Year of 1930," *American Journal of Public Health* 21 (April 1931): 430–31. Inland Steel's company town in Wheelwright, Kentucky, provides another example of the superior living conditions offered by captive mines. Arthur L. Donovan, "Health and Safety in Underground Coal Mining, 1900–1969: Professional Conduct in a Peripheral Industry," in *The Health and Safety of Workers: Case Studies in the Politics of Professional Ethics,* ed. Ronald Bayer (New York: Oxford University Press, 1988), 121–22.

77. Ibid., 122.

78. David, 242.

79. U.S. Department of the Interior, Bureau of Mines, *Minerals Yearbook* (Washington D.C.: GPO, 1950, 1975). John L. Lewis noted that the increasing concentration also had ramifications for the dynamics of industrial relations. Lewis stated, "The mergers of coal properties have produced better leadership on the side of the industry. When we had 11,000 producing entities in the coal industry, no operator could speak for the industry as a whole, on legislation, on wages, or anything. They were all competitive enemies, and acted accordingly. Now the big companies give national leadership to the industry side." "More Machines, Fewer Men—A Union That's Happy About It," *U.S. News and World Report* 47 (9 November 1959): 64.

80. Lewis assumed that older miners displaced by machines would retire on pensions and Social Security while the younger miners who were laid off would find work in the industrialized cities of the north. Dubofsky and Van Tine, 503. Lewis told *U.S. News and World Report,* "It's true there aren't as many miners. But those young men who have been absorbed in other industries are better off than working in a coal mine far underground." "More Machines, Fewer Men," 64. For a description of older miners' reevaluation of this decision in 1973, see Office of Technology Assessment, 130–31.

81. John L. Lewis, Address at the Dedication of the 10 Miners Memorial Hospitals, 2 June 1956, Fund Archives.

CHAPTER THREE

1. Asa Barnes, "Informational Report for 1953—Louisville Area Office," memo to William Draper, 1 June 1954, Fund Archives.

2. Ernest Boyd, Thomas Konrad, and Conrad Seipp, "In and Out of the Mainstream: The Miners' Medical Program, 1946–78," *Journal of Public Health Policy* 3 (December 1982): 434.

3. The President's Commission on Coal, 81. Rusk noted that no one had wanted to run for sheriff in this particular part of east Kentucky since previous sheriffs had died of "'lead poisoning' they hadn't gotten from the drinking water." Johnson, the disabled miner, ran on both the republican and democratic tickets and, according to Rusk, "there never was a sheriff who has had the respect of everybody like Johnson." Howard Rusk to Warren Draper, 13 March 1956, 2, Fund Archives.

4. Warren Draper, "Supplement: Severely Handicapped Cases, October 1947–August, 1949," in UMWA Welfare and Retirement Fund, "Statistical Report for August, 1949," Lorin Edgar Kerr papers.

5. UMWA Welfare and Retirement Fund, "Vocational Rehabilitation Services Report, 1956," 2, Lorin Edgar Kerr papers. Ninety-three percent of the beneficiaries were miners, while miners' wives, widows and dependents comprised the remaining beneficiaries. Ibid., Table A-10, 30.

6. Ibid., Tables A-8 and A-9, 29.

7. Ibid., 19.

8. Howard Rusk to Warren Draper, 13 March 1956, 4, Fund Archives.

9. UMWA Office of Research and Statistics, "Statistical Abstract," various years, Fund Archives. Rehabilitation of beneficiaries continued after 1954 as part of the general Fund program. Outlays for the rehabilitation program were probably greater than $4.5 million as this figure does not include resources expended under the "Special Centers" category. During the period from 1950 to 1954, special center fees comprised an additional $11 million.

10. [Albert Deutsch], "The Healing Chain: How the Miners Created a New Pattern of Medical Care," Ms., 47–48, Robert Kaplan papers. This copy of a remarkable unpublished manuscript attributed to the noted historian and journalist Albert Deutsch has been drawn upon as a unique source of commentary from Fund physicians and administrators.

11. Ibid., 42.

12. Barbara Berney, "The Rise and Fall of the UMW Fund," *Southern Exposure* 6 (1978): 97, and Seltzer, 60.

13. Taubenhaus and Penchansky, 165.

14. The Louisville office also served beneficiaries in the Interior Basin mines in western Kentucky and Indiana. In 1963 the Louisville AMO's jurisdiction was changed to contain only those areas corresponding to the Interior Basin. Louisville's former beneficiaries in eastern Kentucky were transferred to the supervision of the Knoxville AMO. The Louisville office was eventually moved to Evansville, Indiana, in the late 1960s.

15. This procedure should not be confused with preadmission review. It was intended only to assure hospitals that they would receive payment for services rendered.

16. Leslie Falk, "Comprehensive Care in Medical Care Programs: The U.M.W.A. Welfare Fund," *Medical Care* 6 (September-October 1968): 403, and Deane Brooke, "Fund Medical Program," memo to Participating Hospitals and Physicians, UMWA District 29, 10 March 1954, Fund Archives.

17. Falk, "Comprehensive Care," 409, and David, 175.

18. T. Parran and L. Falk, "Collective Bargaining for Medical Benefits: A Recent Development in the U.S.A.," *British Journal of Preventive and Social Medicine* 7 (July 1953): 90.

19. Name of physician withheld at the request of the Archives. Letter to William Draper, 21 April 1959, Fund Archives.

20. Taubenhaus and Penchansky, 165. Janet Ploss reported that the Fund solicited a proposal from Blue Cross in exploring avenues to deliver care. However, Blue Cross was unable to provide the scope of care desired by the Fund. For example, Blue Cross, like most commercial insurers, typically excluded care for pre-existing conditions from its policies. Janet Ploss, "A History of the Medical Care Program of the UMWA Welfare and Retirement Fund" (M.A. thesis, Johns Hopkins University, 1981), 51.

21. [Deutsch], 44.

22. Taubenhaus and Penchansky, 168.

23. Warren Draper, "The Medical Care Program of the UMWA Welfare and Retirement Fund," Address to the New England Hospital Assembly, Boston, 25 March 1958, 6, Robert Kaplan papers.

24. The President's Commission on Coal, 82–83.

25. Taubenhaus and Penchansky, 168.

26. The President's Commission on Coal, 82–83.

27. [Deutsch], 43.

28. The Fund provided coverage for primary care to "grant" beneficiaries only. These were beneficiaries who also were receiving other subsidies from the Fund—pensioners, disabled beneficiaries, and widows. Grant beneficiaries probably received this coverage because they lacked access to check-off plans for primary care.

29. This problem was compounded when, in some instances, miners were found to be lending their health cards to friends and relatives not covered by the plan. The President's Commission on Coal, 82.

30. Taubenhaus and Penchansky, 167.

31. A separate study compiled by the Fund in 1952 corroborates these findings for the period before 1955. The Fund found that in 1952, Fund beneficiaries made up 27.2 percent of all cases in West Virginia; 12.4 percent of patient days and 18.1 percent of cases in Kentucky; 6.1 percent of days and 5.1 percent of cases in Alabama; and 3.6 percent of days and 3.1 percent of cases in Pennsylvania. UMWA Welfare and Retirement Fund, "Hospital and Physicians Service Report, 1952," 3–4, Lorin Edgar Kerr papers. The Fund also found that in the first quarter of 1952, 82.6 percent of all hospitals in West Virginia served Fund beneficiaries, 50.0 percent in Kentucky, 23.6 percent in Alabama, and 32.3 percent in Pennsylvania. UMWA Welfare and Retirement Fund, "Volume of Hospital Service and Type of Hospital Providing It," November 1952, Lorin Edgar Kerr papers.

32. Throughout the United States in 1959, 73 hospitals (excluding the Fund's own Miners Memorial Hospitals) had a patient base that was made up of at least 10 percent Fund beneficiaries. While this number of hospitals declined over time, by 1971, 89 hospitals still had 5 percent or more of their patient base comprised of miners and their families. The majority of these hospitals were located in Appalachia. UMWA Welfare and Retirement Fund, Office of Research and Statistics, "1950 Fund Monthly Reports," various years, Fund Archives.

33. The numbers of physicians and hospitals are reported in Taubenhaus and Penchansky, 167. The number of beneficiaries and total cost are reported in Kaplan, 92–103. Fund expenditures on health amounted to only 4.5 percent of its total outlay and represented the lowest category of spending in this period. The greatest percentage of the Fund's total outlay, 61.2 percent or over $64 million, was paid out in disability grants and widows' assistance. Pensions comprised the next largest category, representing over $30 million or 29.0 percent of Fund expenditures while death benefits comprised roughly $5.5 million or 5.3 percent of Fund outlays. Ibid.

34. [Deutsch], 42.

35. It should be noted that the Fund's elimination of coverage for routine care in theory did not in practice eliminate Fund reimbursement for these services. Given the acute shortage of specialists in the coalfields, many general practitioners were able to call themselves "specialists" and the Fund was left with little choice but to reimburse them as such. [Deutsch], 46. This dilemma diminished over time as the Fund managed to recruit more specialists to work in the coalfields.

36. The Fund apparently considered administering the check-off plans itself. In 1952 Warren Draper proposed having beneficiaries pay their check-offs for routine care to the Fund instead of to private practitioners. With these resources, Draper argued that the Fund could provide comprehensive care and reduce unnecessary hospitalization. By paying physicians for home and office care, the Fund would also have greater ability to super-

vise and recruit physicians. Warren Draper, "Tightening Medical Expenditures," memo to Josephine Roche, 20 August 1952, Fund Archives.

37. Roy Penchansky, Beryl Safford, and Henry Simmons, "Medical Practice in a Group Setting: The Russellton Experience," in (ed.) Roy Penchansky, *Health Services Administration: Policy Cases and the Case Method* (Cambridge: Harvard University Press, 1968), 187.

38. Hubert Marshall, "Informational Report for 1953," memo to Warren Draper, 27 April 1954, Fund Archives.

39. Hubert Marshall, "Annual Report for 1954," memo to Warren Draper, 30 June 1955, 14, Fund Archives.

40. Ibid.

41. Ivana Krajcinovic-Sabelli, "The Welfare and Retirement Fund of the United Mine Workers of America: Innovations in Collective Bargaining and the Provision of Health Care" (Ph.D. diss., Yale University, 1993), 267–77.

42. Emphasis in the original. Deane Brooke, "Fund Policy on Home and Office Care," memo to Warren Draper, 26 January 1962, Fund Archives.

43. The check-off plans that predated the Fund had also used reasons of "morality" to preclude coverage for the treatment of alcoholism and venereal disease (see chapter 2).

44. The Fund had covered treatments that were the responsibility of employers due to the difficulties miners faced in recovering these charges from employers (see chapter 2). Changes in the Workmen's Compensation Law and its enforcement eventually reduced these obstacles. Anecdotal evidence suggests that injured miners' chances of recovering medical costs also increased as a result of the help Fund administrators provided in preparing compensation cases.

45. AMOs promoted some outreach efforts aimed at educating beneficiaries in order to reduce excessive utilization. For example, the Johnstown AMO met with an average of 15 beneficiaries per day in its office in order to better explain Fund policies. The AMO also communicated with local union officials about its operations. F. H. Arestad, "Johnstown Area Report," memo to Warren Draper, 1954, 8, Fund Archives. However, there is little evidence of these efforts, suggesting that the AMOs placed more emphasis on influencing the behavior of providers.

46. Warren Draper, "Tightening Medical Expenditures," memo to Josephine Roche, 20 August 1952, 1, Fund Archives.

47. Hubert Marshall, "Informational Report for 1953," memo to Warren Draper, 27 April 1954, 6, Fund Archives.

48. Emphasis added. Ibid., 2, 7.

49. Warren Draper, "Tightening Medical Expenditures," memo to Josephine Roche, 20 August 1952, 1, Fund Archives.

50. Deane Brooke, "Informational Report for 1953," memo to Warren Draper, 1 June 1954, Fund Archives, and Leslie Falk, "Annual Report for 1954," memo to Warren Draper, 14 July 1955, 1, Fund Archives.

51. "Informational Report for 1953—Denver Area," memo to Warren Draper, 1954, Fund Archives.

52. William Riheldaffer, "Informational Report—Charleston Area Office 1953," memo to Warren Draper, 4 May 1954, Fund Archives.

53. "Annual Report, Johnstown Area Medical Office," 15 April 1958, 2, Fund Archives.

54. Warren Draper, "Fund Utilization of Hospital Service," memo to area administrators, 24 January 1956, Fund Archives.

55. Deane Brooke, "Informational Report for 1954," memo to Warren Draper, 28 June 1955, 2, Fund Archives.

56. Allen Koplin, "Annual Report for 1954," memo to Warren Draper, 26 May 1955, 2, Fund Archives.

CHAPTER FOUR

1. Asa Barnes, "Informational Report for 1953—Louisville Area Office," memo to Warren Draper, 1 June 1954, Fund Archives.

2. The Louisville AMO noted, moreover, that two local physicians decided to build a modern 54-bed hospital in the mountains of Prestonburg, Kentucky, based on the guaranteed income for specialist and hospital services provided by the Fund. Ibid.

3. Taubenhaus and Penchansky, 169.

4. Berney, 97.

5. The Fund would later pay the co-insurance on Medicare policies for eligible beneficiaries. Falk, "Comprehensive Care," 409.

6. Warren Draper, "The Medical Care Program of the UMWA Welfare and Retirement Fund," Address to the New England Hospital Assembly, Boston, 25 March 1958, 6, Robert Kaplan papers.

7. F. H. Arestad, "Johnstown Area Report," memo to Warren Draper, 1954, 2–4, Fund Archives.

8. Ibid., 7.

9. Allen Koplin, "Informational Report for 1953," memo to Warren Draper, 28 May 1954, 1, Fund Archives.

10. Hubert Marshall, "Annual Report for 1954," memo to Warren Draper, 30 June 1955, 4, Fund Archives.

11. Asa Barnes, "Informational Report for 1954—Louisville Area Office," memo to Warren Draper, 15 May 1955, 13, Fund Archives.

12. Hubert Marshall, "Annual Report for 1958," memo to Warren Draper, 8 April 1958, 6–7, Fund Archives.

13. Likewise, the Fund also required hospitals to meet standards for accreditation. However, because the shortage of hospitals was even greater than the shortage of physicians in the coalfields, in practice the Fund often had to keep substandard hospitals on its list. The AMOs placed great pressure on these hospitals to improve conditions. John Winebrenner, "Informational Report Summary (1953)," memo to Warren Draper, 1 June 1954, Fund Archives.

14. Taubenhaus and Penchansky, 175. This task often required a substantial amount of the AMOs' attention, especially in areas where the Fund had relatively less influence. In 1954 the Denver AMO devoted *all* of its attention beyond routine billing and operations to its imposition of a professional standards policy. William Dorsey, "Informational Report for 1954—Denver Office," memo to Warren Draper, 6 July 1955, 1–2, Fund Archives. It took the St. Louis AMO nearly three years to shift surgical procedures in its area from general practice surgeons to qualified specialists. George Brother, "Annual Report—1958," memo to Warren Draper, 10 March 1958, 1, Fund Archives. In another attempt to reduce surgery rates, in 1955 the Fund unsuccessfully attempted to institute a preadmission consultation policy that required physicians to consult the Fund or a specialist before admitting a patient to a hospital. When the Fund had experimented with

requiring preadmission consultation with a specialist in one Area, it found that hospital days decreased by 36.8 percent and the volume of surgical procedures decreased by 16.5 percent. However, organized medicine opposed this policy stating that it discriminated against general practitioners and denied patients free choice of physicians. The strength of this opposition forced Draper to withdraw the requirement (see chapter 6). Draper, 7.

15. Warren Draper, "Present Status of Physicians and Hospitals," memo to Josephine Roche, 31 October 1957, Fund Archives.

16. UMWA Welfare and Retirement Fund, *Annual Report* (Washington, D.C.: UMWA, 1958), cited in Taubenhaus and Penchansky, 179.

17. Ibid.

18. Ironically, the Pittsburgh AMO cuts were realized, in part, by boycotts organized by local medical societies. Leslie Falk, "Informational Data from Annual Report of 1958," memo to Warren Draper, 28 March 1958, 1–2, Fund Archives.

19. "Annual Report, 1957, Charleston Area Medical Office," memo to Warren Draper, 25 March 1958, 1, Fund Archives.

20. Hubert Marshall, "Annual Report for 1958," memo to Warren Draper, 8 April 1958, 6, Fund Archives.

21. "Annual Report, Johnstown Area Medical Office," memo to Warren Draper, 15 April 1958, 1, Fund Archives.

22. Office of Research and Statistics, "Statistical Report," various years, Fund Archives.

23. Ibid. Data on expenditure per beneficiary is not available for the period after 1965.

24. If the expenditures associated with the Miners Memorial Hospital Association are excluded, the savings to the Fund from 1957 to 1958 are even greater. Here, overall expenditure per beneficiary decreased 5.8 percent, by far the largest decrease in the period for which these data are available.

25. Further evidence of the significance of the initial impact of the policy change and the subsequent decline in its magnitude over time is presented in Krajcinovic-Sabelli, 493–504.

26. The other "important" question was "how organized medicine would react." The reaction of organized medicine was probably only of concern in Pennsylvania at this time. "Annual Report, Johnstown Area Medical Office," memo to Warren Draper, 15 April 1958, 1, Fund Archives.

27. Hubert Marshall, "Annual Report for 1958," memo to Warren Draper, 8 April 1958, 11–12, Fund Archives.

28. Allen N. Koplin, Richard Hutchison, and Bruce K. Johnson, "Influence of a Managing Physician on Multiple Hospital Admissions," *American Journal of Public Health* 49 (September 1959): 1175.

29. Lorin Edgar Kerr, "Desire, Expectation and Reality in a Union Health Program," *The New England Journal of Medicine,* 23 May 1968, 1150–51.

30. "Multiple" was defined as those who made three or more visits a year and ten or more visits in the previous five years.

31. Koplin, Hutchison, and Johnson, 1174–80.

32. "Annual Report, 1957, Charleston Area Medical Office," 25 March 1958, Fund Archives.

33. John Newdorp, "Field Trip to Birmingham and Knoxville, April 26–30, 1964," memo to Warren Draper, 5 May 1964, Fund Archives.

34. The precise number of group practice clinics is difficult to determine, probably due to inconsistencies in terminology. The terms "group practice" and "clinic" are often used

interchangeably, without an indication of whether the term refers to an individual clinic or to a cluster of clinics. For instance, Kerr mentions the existence of a total of 37 clinics in 1968. Kerr, 1151. Newdorp mentions the existence of 31 nonprofit clinics in 1970. John Newdorp, "Clinics," memo to Josephine Roche, 27 May 1970, 3, Fund Archives. Seltzer mentions a system of 50 clinics. Seltzer, 143. Table 8 and Map 2 combine the clinics identified in these sources as well as clinics mentioned in documents in the Fund Archives.

35. Edwin P. Jordan, "Group Practice," *New England Journal of Medicine* 250 (1 April 1954): 558.

36. Penchansky, Safford, and Simmons, 182. The number of group practices rose more rapidly after the AMA ended years of opposition to these arrangements and endorsed group practices in 1959. In 1965 there were 4,289 group practices and by 1969, their number had risen to 6,371. The number of physicians involved in group practices rose from 13,009 in 1959 to 28,381 in 1965, and to 40,093 in 1969. It is important to note, however, that the percentage of prepaid group practices, like those developed by the Fund, remained relatively small. Rosemary Stevens, *American Medicine and the Public Interest* (New Haven: Yale University Press, 1971), 424–25.

37. Kerr, 1151. Nationwide, group practices employed an average of six to seven physicians. Sixty percent of the group practices were located in communities with fewer than 60,000 residents. Jordan, 558.

38. The Fund often covered all clinic costs during the initial period of operation, even though non-beneficiaries were receiving care at the clinics. Administrators felt this arrangement was necessary to start operations, especially in areas experiencing physician shortages. Eventually, administrators found other sources of funding for the clinics in order to reduce Fund expenditures: federal and local payment for mental health services, Medicare and Medicaid. Allen Koplin and Thomas Berret, "Review of Fund Relationships with the Centerville Clinic," memo to Josephine Roche, 27 May 1970, 11, Fund Archives.

39. John Newdorp, "Clinics," memo to Josephine Roche, 27 May 1970, 3, Fund Archives.

40. The Fund considered providers to be "antagonistic" if they rejected some or all of the Fund's approach to payment for services and review of care. Ibid.

41. Early references to the creation of the Russellton Clinic can be found in Falk, "Group Health Plans in Coal Mining Communities," *Journal of Health and Human Behavior* 4 (Spring 1963): 9, and [Deutsch], 79–87. Penchansky, Safford, and Simmons present a detailed description of the clinic's experience up until 1964.

42. The physician had been a company doctor and had left his practice reportedly as a consequence of a "strained relationship with the Union and a dwindling 'check-off'." Falk, "Group Health Plans," 9.

43. Letters between W. A. (Tony) Boyle, Lorin Edgar Kerr, Josephine Roche, and Oakwood miners, 1969, Lorin Edgar Kerr papers.

44. Falk, "Group Health Plans," 13.

45. This administrative structure included many of the recommendations of the Boone Report although it is unclear whether the Fund explicitly referred to the report in devising the structure.

46. Falk, "Group Health Plans," 8.

47. Ibid., 10.

48. Boyd, Konrad, and Seipp, 438.

49. Ibid.

50. After the creation of the Miners Memorial Hospitals, the AMOs developed group practices in some areas to act as feeder clinics for the hospitals. William

Riheldaffer, "Medical Management—May, 1963," memo to Warren Draper, 6 June 1963, Fund Archives.

51. The group practices typically offered check-off plans for primary care coverage. In fact, they were more likely to offer such coverage than were solo practitioners.

52. Falk, "Comprehensive Care," 406.

53. John Newdorp, "Clinics," memo to Josephine Roche, 27 May 1970, 2, Fund Archives. Physicians often resisted employing auxiliary personnel because of the substitution effects that subsequently reduce the demand for physician services. In the coalfields, however, the high demand for physician services allayed physicians' concerns over the possible consequences of substitution effects.

54. Robert Zobel, "Clinic Development in the Charleston Area," memo to John Newdorp, 13 February 1973, Lorin Edgar Kerr papers.

55. John Newdorp, "Clinics," memo to Josephine Roche, 27 May 1970, 4, Fund Archives.

56. The literature on peer review suggests that it is not always effective in reducing inappropriate care. However, the physicians employed by the group practices serving Fund beneficiaries were likely to be more affected by peer review than the average physician, given that they subscribed to Fund practices of review.

57. [Deutsch], 9.

58. Penchansky, Safford, and Simmons, 199.

59. Falk, "Group Health Plans," 13. In fact, Falk (the Pittsburgh area medical administrator) himself was an adjunct associate professor of medical and hospital administration at the University of Pittsburgh Graduate School of Public Health.

60. Penchansky, Safford, and Simmons, 195.

61. E. Richard Weinerman, "Report of a Survey of the Group Medical Clinics Serving Beneficiaries of the United Mine Workers Welfare and Retirement Fund in the Pittsburgh Area," 12–17 October 1959, 10, Fund Archives.

62. Ibid.

63. Allen Koplin and Thomas Berret, "Review of Fund Relationships with the Centerville Clinic," memo to Josephine Roche, 27 May 1970, 13–15, Fund Archives.

64. John Newdorp, "Clinics," memo to Josephine Roche, 27 May 1970, 2, Fund Archives.

65. Falk, "Group Health Plans," 13.

66. One-third of the clinics were affiliated with hospitals and physicians at independent clinics typically had admitting privileges at nearby hospitals. Kerr, 1151.

67. Leslie Falk, "Medical Care Program of the UMWA Welfare and Retirement Fund," *Bulletin of the Allegheny County Medical Society,* cited in Kerr, 1152.

68. However, it should be noted that these figures do not control for possible difference in the health needs of the two populations. For example, it may be that self-selection caused relatively healthier patients to use group practices.

69. Penchansky, Safford, and Simmons, 194–95.

70. Leslie Falk, "Informational Report for 1953, Pittsburgh Area," memo to Warren Draper, 5 August 1954, 3, Fund Archives.

71. Krajcinovic-Sabelli, 396–409.

72. John Winebrenner, "Annual Report—1958," memo to Warren Draper, 18 March 1956, 10–13, Fund Archives.

73. Ibid., 11.

74. Eighty-five percent of the Kentucky local's members opted for this coverage and 100 percent of the Virginia locals' members purchased this coverage.

75. The report fails to note that while overall the age distributions were fairly similar, the Virginia locals had a significantly higher percentage of beneficiaries in the child-bearing age group of 15–29. This could, in part, account for higher rates of admissions and lower lengths-of-stay (see chapter 6).

76. Cecil Sharp, "Informational Report for 1953 for St. Louis Area Office," memo to Warren Draper, 4 May 1954, Fund Archives.

77. E. Richard Weinerman, "Report of a Survey of the Group Medical Clinics Serving Beneficiaries of the United Mine Workers Welfare and Retirement Fund in the Pittsburgh Area," 12–17 October 1959, 6–7, Fund Archives.

78. While retainer payments may have been relatively unknown in mainstream medical circles, they were more familiar to the reformers of the coalfields' system of care. For example, the Boone Report had granted high marks to fee-for-time reimbursement. In addition, railroad companies used retainer payments to reimburse their company physicians, a group of approximately 8,000 physicians. Local and state health departments, welfare departments, and nonprofit organizations like the National Foundation for Infantile Paralysis also typically paid physicians on a part-time basis for the time spent with eligible patients. Some large self-insured companies retained physicians to care for workers' compensation cases. Lorin Kerr, "Methods of Paying Physicians," memo to Warren Draper, 4 April 1956, 2–3, Fund Archives.

79. Falk, "Comprehensive Care," 407.

80. Stevens, 424. Stevens notes that group practices were located primarily in the Middle Atlantic, South Atlantic, and Pacific Census Divisions. While Stevens does not identify the practices by name, judging by the geographic areas cited, it is reasonable to assume that the Kaiser Foundation (operating on the west coast) and the UMWA Fund supported a sizable number of these practices.

81. Kerr, 1151.

82. Allen Koplin and Thomas Berret, "Review of Fund Relationships with the Centerville Clinic," memo to Josephine Roche, 27 May 1970, Fund Archives.

83. Ibid., 8.

84. Allen Koplin, "Retainer Payments for Physicians' Services," *American Journal of Public Health* 57 (August 1967): 1368.

85. Hubert Marshall, "Informational Report for 1953," memo to Warren Draper, 27 April 1954, 2, Fund Archives.

86. For example, in 1954, the Birmingham AMO used a full-time net equivalent physician income of $20,000 to compute physician retainers. Allen Koplin, "Informational Report for 1953," memo to Warren Draper, 28 May 1954, 3, Fund Archives.

87. Kerr, 1150, and Taubenhaus and Penchansky, 166.

88. Ploss, 74–75.

89. Kerr, 1151.

90. Falk, "Group Health Plans," 11–12.

91. Fee-for-service patients included both those on public assistance and private patients. Penchansky, Safford, and Simmons, 187.

92. Leslie Falk, "Method of Payment for Medical Services to Beneficiaries of the UMWA Welfare and Retirement Fund," *The Pennsylvania Medical Journal* 58 (May 1955): 465.

93. Koplin, 1365.

94. Newdorp, "Clinics," memo to Josephine Roche, 27 May 1970, 5, Fund Archives.

95. Penchansky, Safford, and Simmons, 186–88. These figures provide only a rough measure of cross-subsidization for two reasons. First, the percentages presented are based on approximate data on the number of patients and amount of payments. Second,

Penchansky, Safford, and Simmons do not indicate the relative intensity of the use of physician services by the two groups. More broadly, however, there is little other evidence to suggest that the cross-subsidization was a problem. For example, an in-depth study of the Centerville Clinic did not reveal cross-subsidization. Allen Koplin and Thomas Berret, "Review of Fund Relationships with the Centerville Clinic," memo to Josephine Roche, 27 May 1970, 12, Fund Archives.

96. The success of this argument requires that the fees paid by non-beneficiaries are greater than or equal to the clinic's variable costs. Newdorp does not mention whether this was generally the case. John Newdorp, "Clinics," memo to Josephine Roche, 27 May 1970, Fund Archives.

97. Ibid., 5.

98. Kerr, 1151.

99. It is important to remember that retainer payments were made to physicians providing specialist care in offices and hospitals. They should not be confused with retainer payments to general practitioners—like capitation payments to physicians in HMOs—which further reduce the incentives for unnecessary specialist care.

100. A more detailed description of the number and type of providers participating in the program in the Beckley AMO is presented in Krajcinovic-Sabelli, 505–9.

101. Office of Research and Statistics, "Summary of Retainers," various years, Fund Archives.

102. The trend of surgical cases largely resembles, not surprisingly, the pattern of hospital calls. Retainer physicians performed only 4,913 surgeries in 1953, the first year that these data are available. The number of surgeries performed by retainer physicians quickly rose to an average of approximately 24,000 surgeries per year in the period from 1957 to 1965. It is interesting to note that the eligibility cuts of mid-1960 (see chapter 6) were probably responsible, in large part, for the dramatic decline in surgeries performed by retainer physicians from 28,872 in 1960 to 13,431 in 1962. UMWA Office of Research and Statistics, "Statistical Reports," various years, Fund Archives.

103. If the number of beneficiaries cared for by retainer physicians increased during this period, then the rate of calls per beneficiary actually fell during this period.

104. For additional evidence suggesting that the use of retainer payments was effective in decreasing the hospital discharge rate, see Krajcinovic-Sabelli, 493–504.

105. For a more detailed examination of the regional variation in use of retainer payments, see Krajcinovic-Sabelli, 431–46.

106. "Comparison of Volume and Cost of Service by Physicians Paid on Retainer and Fee-for-Service Basis in the Pittsburgh Area," undated report, Fund Archives. The results of this survey should be interpreted with caution since the survey assumes that there were no differences in the relative severity of illness between patients treated by retainer physicians and those treated by fee-for-service physicians.

107. However, without a standard for the appropriate number of calls, it is impossible to determine whether fee-for-service physicians provided too much service or retainer physicians provided too little service.

108. Retainer physicians received an even greater share of the payments for outpatient care: in 1955 they received 19 percent of outpatient care payments and in 1956 they received 67 percent of outpatient care payments. "Pittsburgh Area: Payments for Physicians' Services," undated table, Fund Archives.

109. At the start of the program in 1953, the standard fees were $7.40 per hospital visit and $5.16 per office visit. By 1962, the standard fees had reached $12.00 per hospital visit and $8.00 per office visit.

110. UMWA Office of Research and Statistics, "Summary of Retainers," various years, Fund Archives.

111. The change in reporting format probably was prompted by the inception of Medicare in July of 1966. Thereafter, Medicare payments were analyzed separately from Fund payments.

112. William H. Anderson, M.D., to Lorin Edgar Kerr, 4 June 1968, Lorin Edgar Kerr papers.

CHAPTER FIVE

1. Warren Draper, "Review of Memorial Hospital Budgets by Committee Appointed by the Executive Medical Officer," memo to John Morrison, 13 May 1957, Fund Archives.

2. Warren Draper, John Newdorp, and John Morrison, "Statement by Officers of the Medical Service of the UMWA Welfare and Retirement Fund Concerning Necessity of Additional Hospital Facilities in Coal Mining Areas," address to the Trustees of the Welfare and Retirement Fund, 8 October 1951, Robert Kaplan papers. Data from the first quarter of 1952 revealed that while only 6.4 percent of all admissions in the United States were to proprietary hospitals, 33.4 percent of Fund beneficiaries were treated at proprietary hospitals. Conversely, the proportion of Fund beneficiaries admitted to nonprofit hospitals, 56.6 percent, was below the national average of 68.0 percent of admissions to nonprofit hospitals. Finally, 25.6 percent of U.S. patients were admitted to government hospitals while only 10.0 percent of Fund beneficiaries were treated in government hospitals. UMWA Welfare and Retirement Fund, "Volume of Hospital Service and Type of Hospital Providing It," November 1952, Lorin Edgar Kerr papers.

3. Warren Draper, John Newdorp, and John Morrison, "Review of Memorial Hospital Budgets."

4. Ibid. Lack of admitting privileges also hampered the Fund's ability to develop group practices. In 1954 Beckley administrators noted, "Since all hospitals are privately owned and with closed staffs, it is impossible to develop outside groups [practices] due to lack of hospital privileges. It is hoped that the new UMWA Beckley Memorial Hospital will offer possibilities for renewing efforts to develop group practice clinics." Deane Brooke, "Informational Report for 1953," memo to Warren Draper, 1 June 1954, Fund Archives.

5. [Deutsch], 58.

6. Draper, Newdorp, and Morrison, "Statement by Officers of the Medical Service."

7. [Deutsch], 59.

8. The Fund failed to obtain Hill-Burton funds for the construction of the hospitals. The state Hospital Commissions which allocated these funds typically had a number of owners of for-profit hospitals in their ranks who opposed granting monies to the Fund for the construction of hospitals that would compete with their own. Draper, Newdorp, and Morrison, "Statement by Officers of the Medical Service."

9. After his tenure with the MMHA, Mott became head of the Community Health Association in Detroit, a labor-community plan sponsored by the United Auto Workers. [Deutsch], 60.

10. The MMHA chain stretched 250 miles. The central hospitals were the largest: 207 beds at Beckley, 203 at Harlan, and 153 at Williamson. The community hospitals were smaller: 94 beds at Whitesburg, 87 at Man, 86 at Hazard, 79 at Middlesboro, 62 at McDowell, 62 at Wise, and 52 at Pikeville.

11. By 1963, the hospitals in Hazard, McDowell, Middlesboro, and Whitesburg provided 42 percent of the total beds in this region of Kentucky. "Appalachian Regional Hospitals Mark Fifth Anniversary of Service in High Quality Care to Three-State Area," *Group Health and Welfare News* September 1968: 4.

12. The Man, Pikeville, and McDowell Memorial Hospitals acted as satellites for the central hospital at Williamson; the Hazard, Whitesburg, Wise, and Middlesboro Memorial Hospitals acted as satellites for the central hospital at Harlan; and the central hospital at Beckley acted on its own without satellites.

13. The budgets had some flexibility and additional funds could be obtained through discussions with the relevant AMO. MMHA, Budget Committee, "Report of the Budget Committee," 13 June 1957, 2, Fund Archives.

14. Ibid., 1.

15. Asa Barnes, Deane Brooke, William Riheldaffer, and John Winebrenner, "Utilization of MMHA Hospitals," memo to Warren Draper, 2 December 1958, Fund Archives.

16. Warren Draper, "Utilization of MMHA Hospitals," memo to John Newdorp, 15 September 1958, Fund Archives.

17. The Fund also made arrangements for the clinics to accept the prepayment plans for routine care that local mining families carried. MMHA, Budget Committee, "Report of the Budget Committee," 13 June 1957, Fund Archives.

18. Dr. Diessner, "Utilization of this Hospital by Beneficiaries," memo to John Newdorp, 31 October 1958, Fund Archives.

19. A.H. Robinson, "Utilization of Miners Memorial Hospitals," memo to John Newdorp, 14 November 1958, Fund Archives.

20. John Newdorp, "Utilization of Miners Memorial Hospitals," memo to A.H. Robinson, 5 December 1958, Fund Archives.

21. John Newdorp, untitled memo to J. Huston Westover, 17 October 1958, Fund Archives.

22. [Deutsch], 9.

23. John Newdorp, untitled memo to Warren Draper, 18 December 1958, Fund Archives.

24. [Deutsch], 72–73.

25. Warren Draper, "Review of Memorial Hospital Budgets by Committee Appointed by the Executive Medical Officer," memo to John Morrison, 13 May 1957, Fund Archives.

26. [Deutsch], 66–68.

27. Ibid., 70–71.

28. Josephine Roche, untitled memo to Warren Draper et al., 17 February 1959, Fund Archives.

29. Warren Draper, "Review of Memorial Hospital Budgets."

30. [Deutsch], 70.

31. Warren Draper, "Review of Memorial Hospital Budgets."

32. [Deutsch], 7.

33. Streit rejected the notion that the MMHA hospitals produced reductions in overall hospital admission rates. Dr. Streit, "Your Questionnaire *Re* Utilization of Hospitals," memo to Warren Draper, 26 October 1961, Fund Archives. Regression analysis demonstrates that the presence of the Memorial Hospitals did not, in fact, reduce discharge rates in the areas where they operated. Krajcinovic-Sabelli, 493–504. By contrast, the Kaiser

Foundation built and operated its hospitals to allow its program to reap savings from better coordination between care provided in various settings.

34. Drs. Overholt and Arestad, "Report on Visits to Miners' Hospitals," 1957, 2–3, Fund Archives. However, Newdorp later argued that the Memorial Hospitals' costs were actually lower than the national average when certain adjustments were made. Specifically, Newdorp argued that for the comparison to be fair, the estimated cost of outpatient departments should be subtracted from MMHA figures as these costs were excluded from the national figures. John Newdorp to John Morrison, 22 June 1962, 1, Fund Archives.

35. Deane Brooke, "Informational Report on Activities of the Beckley Area Medical Office for the Past Year," memo to Warren Draper, 11 March 1958, Fund Archives. These figures do not account for the fact that the Memorial Hospitals typically provided care for relatively more serious cases.

36. Krajcinovic-Sabelli, 462–76.

37. The Beckley Memorial Hospital lacked room to care for additional beneficiaries due to occupancy by non-beneficiaries and a failure to transfer eligible patients. John Newdorp, draft memo to Dr. Wilder, 24 January 1962, attached to Warren Draper, "Utilization of Memorial Hospitals," memo to John Newdorp, 21 January 1962, Fund Archives.

38. UMWA Welfare and Retirement Fund, Office of Research and Statistics, "Hospital Statistics—Most Frequently Used," annual statistical reports, Fund Archives.

39. John Newdorp to John Morrison, 22 June 1962, Fund Archives.

40. This debate can be seen in the numerous memos found in the Fund Archives prepared by members of the MMHA's Budget Committee in reference to the text of the 1957–58 MMHA Budget Report.

41. Dr. Riheldaffer, "Budget—MMHA—1959–60," memo to Warren Draper, 21 April 1959, Fund Archives.

42. John Newdorp, written answers to questions submitted by Fred Luigart of the *Courier-Journal,* Hazard, Kentucky, attached to John Newdorp to Harold Ward, 15 December 1961, Fund Archives.

43. UMWA Welfare and Retirement Fund, Office of Research and Statistics, "Hospital Statistics—Most Frequently Used," annual statistical reports, Fund Archives.

44. Deane Brooke, "Informational Report on Activities of the Beckley Area Medical Office for the Past Year," memo to Warren Draper, 11 March 1958, Fund Archives.

45. A more detailed examination of the significance of this phenomenon is presented in Krajcinovic-Sabelli, 394–406.

46. John Newdorp, written answers to questions submitted by Fred Luigart of the *Courier-Journal,* Hazard, Kentucky, attached to John Newdorp to Harold Ward, 15 December 1961, Fund Archives.

47. [Deutsch], 7.

48. Ibid., 14–15.

49. Ibid.

50. Finley, 186.

51. Ibid., 186–87.

CHAPTER SIX

1. [Deutsch], 49–50, 56.

2. Berney, 98.

3. Taubenhaus and Penchansky, 171.

4. Berney, 98.

5. American Medical Association, Council on Medical Service, *Report of the Fourth Conference on Medical Care in the Bituminous Coal Mine Area,* Charleston, West Virginia, 6 May 1956, 28, reprinted in M. L. Ingebar, "The Medical, Health and Hospital Service of the Welfare and Retirement Fund," Ms, November 1958, Robert Kaplan papers.

6. Taubenhaus and Penchansky, 177–81.

7. Ibid., 175–76.

8. Despite these reservations, the administrator continued to favor Fund efforts to improve relations with organized medicine: "And yet, organizations such as the Fund without doubt will gain far more if they can secure the cooperation of physicians themselves in policing unsavory members than they will gain in attempting unilateral action against such physicians. 'Getting tough' with physicians is essentially the wrong approach to the problem and should be used only as a last resort. Repeated efforts at cooperation with various organized groups of medicine are favored." Warren Draper, "Comments by Dr. Streit on Physician Relationships" (attachment), memo to Area Administrators, 19 May 1954, Fund Archives.

9. Warren F. Draper, "The Medical Care Program of the UMWA Welfare and Retirement Fund," *Journal of the American Medical Association* 172 (2 January 1960): 6.

10. Beryl M. Safford, "Changing a Community's Pattern of Medical Care: The Russellton Experience," in (ed.) R. Penchansky, *Health Services Administration: Policy Cases and the Case Method* (Cambridge: Harvard University Press, 1968), 258. The physician finally obtained admitting privileges after winning an antitrust suit. Berney, 98.

11. Safford, 224.

12. Berney, 98.

13. Draper, 36.

14. Safford, 242.

15. American Medical Association, Council on Medical Service, 28.

16. [Deutsch], 5.

17. Ibid., 98.

18. Ibid., 5.

19. Letter to Leslie Falk, 24 February 1958, Fund Archives. The name of the physician has been withheld at the request of the Archives.

20. Draper, 36.

21. [Deutsch], 94.

22. American Medical Association, Council on Medical Service, 28.

23. Department of Energy, Energy Information Administration, *Coal Data: A Reference* (Washington, D.C.: GPO, 1982), Table 8, 37.

24. Nonunion operators could lower their costs by paying lower wages, especially after mechanization increased the supply of unemployed miners. They could reap additional savings by avoiding royalty payments to the Fund. The 40-cent royalty represented roughly 8.3 percent of the price of coal in the 1950s.

25. U.S. Department of Energy, Energy Information Administration, Table 6, 32.

26. U.S. Department of the Interior, Bureau of Mines, *Mineral Yearbook.*

27. U.S. Department of Labor, Bureau of Labor Statistics, *Technology, Production, and Labor in the Bituminous Coal Industry, 1950–1979,* by Rose Zeisel et al., Bulletin 2072 (Washington, D.C.: GPO, 1981), Table 2, 4.

28. Ibid., Table 41, 58. Net worth is defined as the sum of common and preferred stocks, surplus reserves, paid-in surplus, earned surplus, and undivided profits.

29. Seltzer, 86.

30. Office of Technology Assessment, 133.

31. "Return" is defined as net profits as a percentage of invested capital. No figures on return are available for 1955. "Fortune 500," *Fortune,* July 1955, July 1960, and July 1965.

32. In 1976, between 90 to 94 percent of underground miners worked under union contracts while only 60 to 64 percent of surface miners worked under collective bargaining agreements. U.S. Department of Labor, Bureau of Labor Statistics, 66. Since surface mining operations were more productive, they could afford to pay their workers higher wages in order to prevent unionization. Furthermore, since surface mining operations were relatively new and often located in regions outside of those that had been organized, their workforces had fewer historic ties to the union.

33. Navarro, 228.

34. Office of Technology Assessment, 126.

35. By 1964, in part because of the work of the Fund, miners' life expectancy had increased to 73 years, above the U.S. average of 69. David, 169–72.

36. The aging of the beneficiary pool increased over time as emigrants from the coalfields tended to be younger workers. Asa Barnes, "Informational Report for 1954—Louisville Area Office," memo to Warren Draper, 15 May 1955, 3, Fund Archives.

37. Office of Research and Statistics, "Statistical Report," various years, Fund Archives. The aging of the Fund's beneficiary pool could also be seen in the growth in the ranks of retired miners. The number of beneficiaries receiving pensions almost doubled during the 1950s to reach a level between 65,000 and 67,000 in the early 1960s. UMWA Welfare and Retirement Fund, *Annual Reports,* various years. By 1965, pensioners and their beneficiaries accounted for 34.8 percent of all Fund expenditures on medical care. Office of Research and Statistics, "Statistical Report," 1965, Fund Archives.

38. The same regional pattern of aging is evident in examining the proportions of hospital admissions by age group. Krajcinovic-Sabelli, 308–11.

39. Office of Technology Assessment, 132, and David, 127–35.

40. The President's Commission on Coal, 110. The 4.6 percent increase in the fatality rate from 1946 to 1960 represented 12 additional deaths. The 21.2 percent increase in the fatality rate from 1960 to 1968 represented 54 additional deaths. The 1968 fatality rate was 26.9 percent higher than the 1946 rate, translating into 65 additional deaths.

41. Curtis Seltzer, "Moral Dimensions of Occupational Health: The Case of the 1969 Coal Mine Health and Safety Act," in (ed.) Ronald Bayer, *The Health and Safety of Workers: Case Studies in the Politics of Professional Ethics* (New York: Oxford University Press, 1988), 247. "Black lung" is a term that describes the stages of respiratory impairment that ultimately lead to coal workers' pneumoconiosis. Textile workers experienced a similar rise in the incidence of respiratory disease—termed "brown lung"—as a result of increased dust levels spawned by the introduction of mechanization in both the cotton fields and in the textile mills. Bennett Judkins, *We Offer Ourselves as Evidence: Toward Workers' Control of Occupational Health* (New York: Greenwood Press, 1986), 41–42.

42. Office of Technology Assessment, 276–78.

43. Since these figures do not include retired or disabled miners, they probably understate the prevalence of the disease. Ibid., 264.

44. Brit Hume, *Death and the Mines: Rebellion and Murder in the United Mine Workers* (New York: Grossman Publishers, 1971), 33.

45. Warren Draper, "Tightening Medical Expenditures," memo to Josephine Roche, 20 August 1952, 2–3, Fund Archives.

46. Miners were allowed to retire at or after age 60 but only those who retired after May 26, 1946, were eligible for pensions. Disabled miners received health benefits for four years subsequent to their last employment and became eligible for health benefits when they received pensions.

47. Finley, 190.

48. Between 1946 and 1952, 32,026 miners had died and left survivors who were eligible for benefits. UMWA Office of Research and Statistics, "Statistical Abstract," January 1953, Fund Archives.

49. The Fund continued to make grants to cover funeral expenses, and provided modest monthly maintenance subsidies and health care to the beneficiary's family for one year following the miner's death.

50. The precise amount of savings is difficult to estimate due to reporting changes in the Fund's *Annual Reports.* For instance, the monthly maintenance benefits to disabled miners were reported together with the amounts spent on the rehabilitation program.

51. Robert J. Meyers, "Experience of the UMWA Welfare and Retirement Fund," *Industrial and Labor Relations Review* 9 (October 1956): 94.

52. Allen Croyle to John L. Lewis, 1 February 1954, Fund Archives.

53. David, 167. These disabled miners typically also had been unable to receive adequate workmen's compensation.

54. Miners who operated their own mines typically mined little more than a "dog hole" and were among the most destitute of miners. These were miners who would have been unemployed otherwise. This group also included those unemployed miners who had not qualified for pensions after the 1953 requirement took effect.

55. Robert Kaplan, "Number and Percentage of Cancellations on July 1, 1960, Together with Number of 85-HS Holders May 1 and July 1, by District," loose table, 1 July 1960, Fund Archives.

56. This action was designed not so much to cut costs, apparently, but rather to eliminate the competitive advantage small mines gained when they failed to make their royalty payments. The trustees hoped that the wildcat strikes that followed the decision would scare these marginal operators into paying and thereby enhance the competitive position of the large mines with which the UMWA was more closely aligned. Finley, 193, and Hume, 32–33.

57. The October increase from $85 to $100 was made on the grounds that it would not eliminate the Fund's operating surplus. Thomas Ryan, "Increase in Pensions to $100 per month effective October 1, 1965," memo to Josephine Roche, 1 October 1965, Fund Archives. The trustees used the same calculus in 1967 to raise pensions to $115. Ryan calculated that a $15 increase would allow a small surplus to continue while a $20 increase would produce a deficit. Thomas Ryan to Josephine Roche, 4 April 1967, Fund Archives.

58. Dubofsky and Van Tine, 520. It should be noted, however, that the reduction in the retirement age to 55 was welcome in an industry that took such a toll on the health of its workers.

59. Finley estimates that 7,000 working miners had been affected by the ruling. Finley, 193. Despite the reversal, the trustees' 1962 decision was considered so egregious that it was revisited in the heralded class action suit known as *Blankenship* settled in 1972 (see chapter 7). In his decision, Judge Gerhard Gesell condemned the denial of benefits to miners whose operators were delinquent in their royalty payments as a violation of the Fund's own principle of guaranteeing benefits regardless of the actions of employers.

60. Ibid., 191–92.

61. John Newdorp, "Trip to Johnstown, Pittsburgh and Morgantown," memo to File, 22 September 1961, Fund Archives.

62. David, 222.

63. John Newdorp, untitled memo to Warren Draper, 18 December 1958, Fund Archives. Some non-beneficiaries were probably former beneficiaries whose eligibility had been severed as a result of the changes in eligibility rules in the early 1960s.

64. UMWA Welfare and Retirement Fund, Office of Research and Statistics, "Statistical Abstract," various years, Fund Archives.

65. The Fund refused to take bids from individual physicians in order to avoid transforming the hospitals into proprietary institutions. Taubenhaus and Penchansky, 174.

66. Dubofsky and Van Tine, 519.

67. As of 1968, the Fund provided about 75 percent of the hospital income. Taubenhaus and Penchansky, 174.

68. Dubofsky and Van Tine, 506–510. Lewis placed the union's funds in highly liquid assets in order to finance these ventures. The union held vast sums of its monies in non-interest-bearing checking accounts: $30 million in 1956 (23 percent of its resources), $14 million in 1961 (14 percent of its resources), $50 million in 1966 (34 percent of its resources), and $75 million in 1967 (44 percent of its resources). David, Table 50, 196. This practice would be condemned in the *Blankenship* decision.

69. Dubofsky and Van Tine, 502.

70. Ibid., 505.

71. Navarro, 221.

72. By 1970, the 40-cent royalty was worth roughly 23 cents in real terms. The UMWA did manage to bargain for higher wages during this period, but the rank-and-file were more concerned with benefits and seniority language than with increased earnings. Lewis's successor, Tony Boyle, also refused to negotiate the seniority provisions that were universally demanded by the rank-and-file. Seltzer, *Fire in the Hole,* 87–88.

73. Dubofsky and Van Tine, 508.

74. Towers, Perrin, Forster, & Crosby, Inc., Preliminary Report, 6 November 1947, Fund Archives.

75. David, 194.

76. Judkins, 76, and Seltzer, "Moral Dimensions," 248.

CHAPTER SEVEN

1. Navarro, Table 2, 228.

2. The reasons for the decline in productivity are unknown but some analysts speculate that the changes in production methods mandated by the Federal Coal Mine Health and Safety Act of 1969 may have contributed to the decline. Navarro, 221.

3. Office of Technology Assessment, 123.

4. U.S. Department of Labor, Bureau of Labor Statistics, 41.

5. For a fuller discussion on the events of the late 1960s and early 1970s, see Seltzer, *Fire in the Hole,* Finley, and Hume.

6. Berney, 100. For a fuller discussion of the operation of the Fund under Huge and Danziger, see Ploss, 113–60.

7. Daniel Marschall, "The Miners and the UMW: Crisis in the Reform Process," *Socialist Review* 40/41 (July–October 1978): 101.

8. Berney, 100.

9. Ibid., 101.

10. Seltzer, 144.

11. Ibid.

12. In most other respects, the 1974 contract was considered to be excellent. High industry profits provided the highest wage increases ever, as well as the inclusion of a cost-of-living escalator and paid sick leave for the first time. Safety language was also strengthened considerably.

13. The separation of funds for health benefits and pensions was prompted by the passage of the Employee Retirement Insurance Security Act (ERISA) which required negotiated pension funds to be fully funded, vested, and guaranteed. The UMWA would no longer be able to alter the level of pensions in order to absorb the high costs of providing medical care. Ploss, 166.

14. Navarro, 223.

15. Organizing in these areas already was complicated by the fact many of these nonunion operators gave their miners the cash equivalent of payments to the Fund in order to deter unionization. Berney, 101.

16. George Getschow, a reporter for the *Wall Street Journal,* calculated that the income lost from wildcat strikes amounted to only 5 percent of the trusts' total income. The relatively small magnitude of this figure casts doubt upon the validity of assertion by the BCOA and UMWA that the strikes were the main cause of the trusts' insolvency. Moreover, Seltzer maintains that two of the largest wildcats actually were provoked by operators. Seltzer, *Fire in the Hole,* 145.

17. As part of the division of the Fund into the four trusts, the trustees were allowed to reallocate funds among the trusts with the approval of the UMWA and the BCOA. The first reallocation was made in May 1976, when funds from the 1950 Pension Trust were transferred to the 1950 Benefit Trust to meet rising health care costs. In October, the UMWA and the BCOA approved a transfer of $60 million from the reserves of the 1974 Benefit Trust to the other three trusts. This transfer aroused some suspicion since the trustees had requested a transfer for only the 1950 Benefit Trust. By transferring funds to all three trusts, the 1974 Benefit Trust was depleted to a much greater extent than necessary. As a result, working miners were forced to suffer benefit cutbacks in the second half of 1977. Finally, in June 1977, no reallocation was made to stave off a third round of cutbacks. Berney reports that operators angered by wildcat strikes refused to agree a transfer. Berney, 101–2. Seltzer maintains that the trustees did not even bother to ask for another reallocation since the operators "had made it clear" that they would not agree to it. Seltzer, 145.

18. The timing of the policy change further angered beneficiaries as the announcement was made only days after Arnold Miller's close reelection to the UMWA presidency.

19. Ploss, 212.

20. Virginia Gemmell and Jane Ray, *Physician Loss in Central Appalachian Coalfield Hospitals and Clinics,* draft report (Washington, D.C.: Appalachian Regional Commission, 1978), cited in Seltzer, *Fire in the Hole,* 146. The consequences of the switch in payment systems were not lost on beneficiaries who formed the Miners Committee to Save Our Clinics. In addition, 20 clinics banded together to form the Associated Clinics of Appalachia in order to achieve a unified voice. Joyce Goldstein, "Who Will Pay the Bill?" *Southern Exposure* 6 (1978): 91.

21. Ploss, 186–87.

22. U.S. Department of Labor, Bureau of Labor Statistics, 25.

23. Seltzer, 153–58.

24. Office of Technology Assessment, 139–40.

25. The remainder of the 1977 contract, unlike its immediate predecessor, did not include many gains. Wages were increased only modestly and the gap in pensions was not eliminated. Miners did not receive the right to strike, one of their biggest demands, although they managed to resist employer efforts to install more restrictive "labor stability" measures. Finally, for the first time the UMWA acceded to bonus plans tied to production. These bonus plans were cause for concern as they provided incentives for management and miners to pay less attention to safety in the mines.

26. Seltzer, 165.

Bibliography

American Medical Association, Council on Medical Service. "Union Health Centers, 1958 Survey." *Journal of the American Medical Association* 168 (1 November 1958): 1234–1238.

Banta, H. David, and Samuel J. Bosch. "Organized Labor and the Prepaid Group Practice Movement." *Archives of Environmental Health* 29 (July 1974): 43–49.

Berney, Barbara. "The Rise and Fall of the UMW Fund." *Southern Exposure* 6 (1978): 95–102.

Boyd, Ernest W., Thomas R. Konrad, and Conrad Seipp. "In and Out of the Mainstream: The Miners' Medical Program, 1946–78." *Journal of Public Health Policy* 3 (December 1982): 432–44.

Brandes, Stuart D. *American Welfare Capitalism.* Chicago: University of Chicago Press, 1976.

Bureau of Cooperative Medicine. *Medical Care in Selected Areas of the Appalachian Bituminous Coal Fields.* New York: Bureau of Cooperative Medicine, 1939.

Corbin, David Alan. *Life, Work, and Rebellion in the Coal Fields.* Urbana: The University of Illinois Press, 1981.

David, John Peter. "Earnings, Health, Safety, and Welfare of the Bituminous Coal Miners Since the Encouragement of Mechanization by the UMW of A." Ph.D. diss., University of West Virginia, 1972.

Derickson, Alan. *Workers' Health, Workers' Democracy: The Western Miners' Struggle, 1981–1925.* Ithaca: Cornell University Press, 1988.

——. "Health Security for All? Social Unionism and Universal Health Insurance, 1935–1958." *Journal of American History* 80 (March 1994): 1333–56.

[Deutsch, Albert]. "The Healing Chain: How the Miners Created a New Pattern of Medical Care." Ms. Robert Kaplan papers, Manuscripts and Archives, Yale University, New Haven.

Donovan, Arthur L. "Health and Safety in Underground Coal Mining, 1960–1969: Professional Conduct in a Peripheral Industry." In (ed.) Ronald Bayer, *The Health and Safety of Workers: Case Studies in the Politics of Professional Ethics.* New York: Oxford University Press, 1988.

Draper, Warren F. "The Medical Program of Welfare and Retirement Fund of the United Mine Workers of America." *Journal of the American Medical Association* 172 (2 January 1960): 33–36.

Dubofsky, Melvyn, and Warren Van Tine. *John L. Lewis.* New York: Quadrangle/The New York Times Book Co., 1977.

Falk, Leslie A. "Method of Payment for Medical Services to Beneficiaries of the UMWA Welfare and Retirement Fund." *The Pennsylvania Medical Journal* 58 (May 1955): 464–67.

——. "Group Health Plans in Coal Mining Communities." *Journal of Health and Human Behavior* 4 (Spring 1963): 4–13.

——. "Coal Miners' Prepaid Medical Care in the United States—and Some British Relationships, 1792–1964." *Medical Care* 4 (January 1966): 37–42.

——. "Comprehensive Care in Medical Care Programs: The U.M.W.A. Welfare Fund." *Medical Care* 6 (September–October 1968): 401–11.

Finley, Joseph E. *The Corrupt Kingdom: The Rise and Fall of the United Mine Workers.* New York: Simon and Schuster, 1972.

Ginger, Ray. "Company-Sponsored Welfare Plans in the Anthracite Industry Before 1900." *Bulletin of the Business Historical Society* 27 (June 1953): 112–20.

Goldstein, Joyce. "Who Will Pay the Bill?" *Southern Exposure* 6 (1978): 89–92.

Hoffman, Lily. *The Politics of Knowledge: Activist Movements in Medicine and Planning.* Albany: State University of New York Press, 1989.

Hume, Brit. *Death and the Mines: Rebellion and Murder in the United Mine Workers.* New York: Grossman Publishers, 1971.

Ingebar, M. L. "The Medical, Health and Hospital Service of the Welfare and Retirement Fund." November 1958. Ms. Robert Kaplan papers, Manuscripts and Archives, Yale University, New Haven.

Janis, Lee, and Milton I. Roemer. "Medical Care Plans for Industrial Workers and Their Relationship to Public Health Programs." *American Journal of Public Health* 38 (September 1948): 1245–53.

Jordan, Edwin P. "Group Practice." *New England Journal of Medicine* 250 (1 April 1954): 558–61.

Judkins, Bennett M. *We Offer Ourselves As Evidence: Toward Workers' Control of Occupational Health.* New York: Greenwood Press, 1986.

Kalet, Anna. "Voluntary Health Insurance in New York City." *American Labor Legislation Review* 6 (June 1916): 142–54.

Kaplan, Robert. "The United Mine Workers' Welfare and Retirement Fund: Its Background and History." Ms. Robert Kaplan papers, Manuscripts and Archives, Yale University, New Haven.

Kennedy, James B. "Beneficiary Features of American Trade Unions." Ph.D. diss., Johns Hopkins University, 1907.

Kerr, Lorin. "Desire, Expectation and Reality in a Union Health Program," *The New England Journal of Medicine* 278 (23 May 1968): 1149–53.

Kindel, D. J. "High Lights of the Medical and Health Program of the Consolidation Coal Company, Inc., Year of 1930." *American Journal of Public Health* 21 (April 1931): 430–31.

Koplin, Allen N. "Retainer Payments for Physicians' Services." *American Journal of Public Health* 57 (August 1967): 1363–73.

Koplin, Allen N., Richard Hutchison, and Bruce Johnson. "Influence of a Managing Physician on Multiple Hospital Admissions." *American Journal of Public Health* 49 (September 1959): 1174–80.

Krajcinovic-Sabelli, Ivana. "The Welfare and Retirement Fund of the United Mine Workers of America: Innovations in Collective Bargaining and in the Provision of Health Care." Ph.D. diss., Yale University, 1993.

Lichtenstein, Nelson. *Labor's War at Home: The CIO in World War II.* Cambridge: Cambridge University Press, 1982.

Lubove, Roy. "Workmen's Compensation and the Prerogatives of Voluntarism." *Labor History* 8 (Fall 1967): 254–79.

Marschall, Daniel. "The Miners and the UMW: Crisis in the Reform Process." *Socialist Review* 40/41 (July–October 1978): 65–115.

McAteer, J. Davitt. *Coal Mine Health and Safety*. New York: Praeger Publishers, 1970.

Meyers, Robert J. "Experience of the UMWA Welfare and Retirement Fund." *Industrial and Labor Relations Review* 9 (October 1956): 93–100.

Miller, Donald L., and Richard E. Sharpless. *The Kingdom of Coal: Work Enterprise, and Ethnic Communities in the Mine Fields*. Philadelphia: University of Pennsylvania Press, 1985.

"More Machines, Fewer Men—A Union That's Happy About It." *U.S. News and World Report*, 9 November 1959, 64.

Munts, Raymond. *Bargaining for Health: Labor Unions, Health Insurance, and Medical Care*. Madison: University of Wisconsin Press, 1967.

Navarro, Peter. "Union Bargaining Power in the Coal Industry, 1945–1981." *Industrial and Labor Relations Review* 36 (January 1983): 214–29.

Office of Technology Assessment. *The Direct Use of Coal*. Washington D.C.: GPO, 1979.

Parran, T., and L. Falk. "Collective Bargaining for Medical Care Benefits: A Recent Development in the U.S.A." *British Journal of Preventive and Social Medicine* 7 (July 1953): 87–94.

Penchansky, Roy, Beryl Safford, and Henry Simmons. "Medical Practice in a Group Setting: The Russellton Experience." In (ed.) R. Penchansky, *Health Services Administration: Policy Cases and the Case Method*. Cambridge: Harvard University Press, 1968.

Peterson, Florence, Everett Kassalow, and Jean Nelson. "Health Benefit Programs Established Through Collective Bargaining." *Monthly Labor Review* 61 (August 1945): 191–209.

Ploss, Janet. "A History of the Medical Care Program of the UMWA Welfare and Retirement Fund." M.A. thesis, Johns Hopkins University, 1981.

The President's Commission on Coal. *The American Coal Miner*. Washington, D.C.: GPO, 1980.

Rowe, Evan Keith. "Employee-Benefit Plans Under Collective Bargaining, Mid-1950." *Monthly Labor Review* 72 (February 1951): 156–62.

Safford, Beryl M. "Changing a Community's Pattern of Medical Care: The Russellton Experience." In (ed.) R. Penchansky, *Health Services Administration: Policy Cases and the Case Method*. Cambridge: Harvard University Press, 1968.

Schwartz, Jerome L. "Early History of Prepaid Medical Care Plans." *Bulletin of the History of Medicine* 39 (September–October 1965): 450–75.

Schwieder, Dorothy, Joseph Hraba, and Elmer Schwieder. *Buxton: Work and Racial Equality in a Coal Mining Community*. Ames: Iowa State University Press, 1987.

Seltzer, Curtis. *Fire in the Hole: Miners and Managers in the American Coal Industry*. Lexington: The University of Kentucky, 1985.

——. "Moral Dimensions of Occupational Health: The Case of the 1969 Coal Mine Health and Safety Act." In (ed.) Ronald Bayer, *The Health and Safety of Workers: Case Studies in the Politics of Professional Ethics*. New York: Oxford University Press, 1988.

Simons, John. "The Union Approach to Health and Welfare." *Industrial Relations* 4 (May 1965): 61–76.

Skolnik, Alfred M. "Employee-Benefit Plans: Developments, 1954–63." *Social Security Bulletin* 28 (April 1965): 4–20.

Somers, Herman M., and Anne R. Somers. *Doctors, Patients, and Health Insurance: The Organization and Financing of Medical Care*. Washington, D.C.: The Brookings Institute, 1961.

Starr, Paul. *The Social Transformation of American Medicine*. New York: Basic Books, 1982.

Stevens, Rosemary. *American Medicine and the Public Interest*. New Haven: Yale University Press, 1971.

Taubenhaus, Marjorie, and Penchansky, Roy. "The Medical Care Program of the United Mine Workers Welfare and Retirement Fund." In (ed.) R. Penchansky, *Health Services Administration: Policy Cases and the Case Method*. Cambridge: Harvard University Press, 1968.

Temin, Peter. "An Economic History of American Hospitals." In (ed.) H.E. Frech, *Health Care in America*. San Francisco: Pacific Research Institute for Public Policy, 1988.

U.S. Coal Mines Administration. *A Medical Survey of the Bituminous-Coal Industry*. Washington, D.C.: GPO, 1947.

U.S. Congress. Senate. Subcommittee of the Committee on Education and Labor. *A Resolution to Investigate Violations of the Right of Free Speech and Assembly and Interference with the Right of Labor to Organize and Bargain Collectively*. 75th Cong., 1st Sess., 30 April, 3–5 May 1937, Harlan County.

U.S. Congress. Senate. *Report of the Joint Committee on Labor-Management Relations*. 80th Cong., 2d sess., 1948.

U.S. Department of Energy. Energy Information Administration. *Coal Data: A Reference*. Washington, D.C.: GPO, 1982.

U.S. Department of Health, Education, and Welfare. Public Health Service. Division of Community Health Services. "Medical Care Financing and Utilization," *Health Economics Series* no. 1. Washington, D.C.: GPO, 1962.

U.S. Department of the Interior. U.S. Bureau of Mines. *Injury Experience in Coal Mining*. Washington, D.C.: GPO, 1950–70.

——. *Minerals Yearbook*. Washington, D.C.: GPO, 1945–1980.

U.S. Department of Labor. Bureau of Labor Statistics. *Technology, Production, and Labor in the Bituminous Coal Industry, 1950–79*, by Rose N. Zeisel et al. Bulletin 2072. Washington, D.C.: GPO, 1981.

U.S. Mine Enforcement Safety Administration. *Injury Experience in Coal Mining*. Washington, D.C.: GPO, 1971–75.

U.S. Treasury Department. "A Survey of the Work of Employees' Mutual Benefit Associations." by Dean K. Brundage. *Public Health Reports* 46 (Sept. 4, 1931): 2102–19.

Index

Lewis, John L. (*continued*)
Fund trustee, 37–38, 42, 58, 67, 149, 156–62. *See also* United Mine Workers of America
Love, George, 47

managed care. *See* group practices; Miners Memorial Hospital Association; United Mine Workers of America Welfare and Retirement Fund
Marschall, Daniel, 166
Marshall, Hurbert, 58, 68–69, 72, 96
McGuiness, Aims, 119, 129
A Medical Survey of the Bituminous-Coal Industry. *See* Boone Report
Medicare, 86n38, 157, 164
mental health, 9, 86n38
Miller, Arnold, 166, 169n18
Miners Memorial Hospital Association (MMHA), 48–49, 81n24, 90n50, 107–30, 135–36, 150; coordination of care in, 111–16, 121; cost control in, 120–27, 129; and Fund trustees, 121, 126–29, 156–57; outpatient care in, 111–13, 116–18, 124; provision of care by, in underserved areas, 108–11, 120, 128–30; reimbursement of physicians in, 119–20; research and education in, 116, 119; sale of, 152, 156–58, 161; utilization of, by beneficiaries, 114, 118, 121–27, 129
Miners Committee to Save Our Clinics, 169n20
moral hazard, 61–62
Morrison, John, 58
Mott, Fred, 109
Murray, Thomas, 37–38
mutual benefit associations, 9–10

National Bank of Washington, 158, 160
National Coal Policy Conference (NCPC), 46–47
National Foundation for Infant Paralysis, 56, 94n78
National Health Service Corps, 77
National Institute for Occupational Health and Safety, 147
National Recovery Act, 47

Newdorp, John, 58, 109, 116, 118, 124–25
North American Coal, 136

organized medicine, 11, 77, 79, 82n26, 83, 108, 131–38, 161–62

Perkins, Frances, 29
Permanente hospitals, 53
personnel management, 9
preventive medicine, 5n1. *See also* United Mine Workers of America Welfare and Retirement Fund: preventive care
primary care. *See* United Mine Workers of America Welfare and Retirement Fund: primary care

Riheldaffer, William, 58, 124
Roche, Josephine, 38, 42, 54, 58, 67, 149, 161, 166
routine care. *See* United Mine Workers of America: primary care
Rusk, Howard, 52–54
Russellton Clinic, 68, 86–90, 92–93, 98, 135, 138

Schmidt, Henry, 58, 136, 149, 161
sickness benefits, 8, 10, 12n26
Southern Coal Producers Association, 46
Standard Oil Company of Louisiana, 9
steelworkers, 90, 93

Taft-Hartley Act, 12, 29, 36, 37n56; injunction under, 38, 40–41, 171
Tennessee Valley Authority, 39–40
third-party insurance. *See* commercial insurance
Thomas, Elbert, 22
Truman, Harry, 31, 37, 40–41, 171

United Mine Workers of America (UMWA), 6, 24–25, 165–66; 1945 contract negotiations, 28–29; 1946 contract negotiations, 29–33; 1947 and 1948 contract negotiations, 36–38; 1949 contract negotiations, 38–41; 1950 Benefit Trust, 168–69, 174–75; 1950 contract (Compromise of 1950), 18, 41–49,